PATIENT BEWARE— DOCTOR TAKE CARE!

By
Edward Zebrowski, M.D.

WOODSTOCK BOOKS
Tampa, Florida

PATIENT BEWARE—
DOCTOR TAKE CARE!

Library of Congress Catalog Card Number 94-61243

ISBN 0-9640096-1-7

Manufactured in the United States of America
First Printing 1994

Published by
WOODSTOCK BOOKS
Tampa, Florida

Dedication

To my wife, Elizabeth, and children, Stephen, Jane,
and Edward.

Contents

Preface

This book, for the most part, is a collection of various bits of medical histories culled from 42 years on the "front lines" of Medicine, beginning with basic medical training, and then while practicing as a family physician in a small town in Connecticut. These bits are then molded into episodes that reveal many of the horrible things that can happen to a patient when he or she goes to see a doctor..

The patients are presented not as dull case histories, but as living human beings. And so are the physicians.

This book is not an indictment of the medical profession. The practice of medicine in the United States is on the highest level both technologically and ethically by deeply dedicated, highly-trained physicians, in spite of all the doctor-bashing that has become so popular today. But medical disasters do occur. While medical technology has advanced, the patient-doctor relationship has deteriorated. In the eyes of the government and the insurance companies, doctors are seen as providers and vendors. And nobody wants to pay physicians for listening to patients. In the rush towards the diagnosis and treatment under a monstrous deluge of paper-work, human suffering is overlooked. This, then, becomes a perfect setting for errors, not only technological, but also in physician judgment. And if the doctor happens to be burdened by individual idiosyncrasies, calamity is sure to follow.

The patient too, can contribute to these disasters in many ways as will be seen. Just as a doctor can learn to become a better physician, a patient can learn to become a more knowledgeable and discriminating individual, so the doctor and the patient can work together as a team and arrive at the proper diagnosis and treatment. After reading this book, the lay person should be better equipped to recognize and choose the proper physician to help him. On the other hand, the resident physician or the physician already in practice should be better able to avoid developing into the type of doctor described in some these pages, individuals so infused with their own importance and lofty status, lacking even the smallest amount of humility, that they are destined to create their own problems over and over again.

In each chapter the reader will see clues, some quite obvious, relating to both the physician and the patient. Following each presentation there is a brief discussion of some of the lessons that may be learned.

Except in the specific chapters related to my relatives or those concerning Governor Trumbull or Colonel Teague, the situations, problems, and individuals involved are all composite depictions, created from thousands of bits of information and written with a certain amount of literary license to illustrate specific points. Any resemblance to any institution or to any living or dead individual is purely coincidental.

EZ
Plainville, Connecticut
March, 1994

Acknowledgments

Again, as with my first book, I am deeply indebted to my daughter, Jane, for all the help and constructive criticism she has given me in the preparation of this second book.

And I must mention my two sons, Stephen and Edward, who also helped me immensely, along with my patient wife, Elizabeth, whose devotion has extended over forty years.

Neither can I overlook the support of my sister, Sophie Lynch, who constantly encouraged me in the completion of this manuscript.

I also have to reach back nearly fifty years to my undergraduate days at Dartmouth, to Professor Arthur Dewing and the course he gave in creative writing. It was at Professor Dewing's request that Robert Frost, then Poet-in-Residence in 1948, read two chapters of my first book and gave me great encouragement to continue writing. But it was my brother Stan, 20 years older than I, who ignited the original fire inside of me by his constructive criticism of my first attempt at writing when I was ten. The fires were banked for many years while I was engaged in the practice of medicine, but now are in full flame once again.

Edward Zebrowski, M.D.
March, 1994
Plainville, Connecticut

Chapter One

The Malingerer

"*T*he next patient is John Patterson," Dr. Tim Murphy said, walking briskly past Patterson's bed without looking at him.

"Wait a minute," I said. *"What about Patterson?"*

Patterson was in a corner bed of the large medical ward of the San Francisco hospital where I was scheduled to start my internship. He, like all the other patients, had been watching our progress as we walked from bed to bed, discussing the status of each patient. Naturally, they were all interested in the new intern on the floor. I was supposed to start working the next day, July 1, 1953, but had come in one day early for orientation purposes so that I wouldn't be swamped with work on my first day. Tim Murphy was the old intern and was moving on to a neurosurgical residency.

"John Patterson is a malingerer," Tim said in an irritated voice, "and we haven't bothered with him for the past month. He refuses to walk and if he wants to rot in that bed, that's exactly what we're going to let him do."

Patterson gave me a look that stopped me dead in my tracks. He was a man pleading for help, but not one word left his lips. As I passed his bed I put my hand on his shoulder. He covered my hand with his own.

It took us an hour to complete the rounds. The patients were the typical ones you would expect to see on a medical ward, suffering from a variety of diseases such as uncontrolled diabetes, severe hypertension, disabling angina, peptic ulcers, gall stones, strokes, heart attacks, asthma, and severe rheumatoid arthritis.

When we finished, Tim informed me there were six patients that he hadn't had time to work up. He also imparted the good news that I should expect at least six new patients every day that would keep me busy until midnight the first few weeks. That schedule was enough to make me shudder.

What he told me was true. The next day was a madhouse and I didn't get back to my room until midnight. The following days were no better. I worked up the new patients, kept up with the old, and gradually finished the patients that Tim Murphy hadn't completed.

On morning rounds that first week, the attending physician, Dr. George Milton, deliberately walked by Patterson's bed without saying a word. And we all followed him silently, ignoring Patterson completely. I caught Patterson's eyes briefly, putting a finger to my lips and nodding my head, hoping he would understand that I would spend more time with him soon. That first weekend I was scheduled to be off duty, but I decided to stay in the hospital and start working on Patterson's problem.

So after lunch at one o'clock on Saturday, I dragged a chair over to Patterson's bed and sat down.

"John," I said, "I'm off this weekend and I'm going to spend the next two days working you over. I'm going to listen to what you have to say, examine you thoroughly, and then go over all your records. I think you have been ignored by everybody in this hospital and you and I together are going to put a stop to that."

He took my hand and kissed it.

"Now wait a minute, John," I said. "I'm not the Pope and I haven't done anything for you yet."

"I know that, Doctor. But you're the first person in this hospital who has bothered to treat me like a human being and is willing to listen to me."

He had tears in his eyes.

The history of the illness that he related was simple. He had been in good health until about five weeks before when he slipped on the walkway of a train engine and struck his back against an iron railing. From that moment, he was unable to walk. He was brought to this hospital immediately and examined by an intern who told him there was no significant injury. X-rays of his back were completed within an hour and read as normal. He was unable to walk when he got to the ward and from that moment on he was considered a malingerer. He had been lying in bed since his admission, ignored by everybody, and getting weaker every day. The nurses were especially mean to him since they felt he refused to walk just to aggravate them.

"I feel that I'm rotting away in this bed just like Dr. Murphy said I would. And nobody believes me when I tell them I can't walk."

"I believe you, John," I said. "But tell me, have you tried to walk in physiotherapy?"

"Yes, I have. But I can't stand up. How can you walk if you can't stand up?"

Besides the inability to stand and walk, he complained of numbness and tingling in his lower extremities.

On physical examination, I found only one abnormality, one that I had never seen before in any other patient, and that was an extremely unusual Babinski reflex. The Babinski reflex is elicited by scraping the lateral aspect of the sole of the foot. It is considered positive if the big toe moves upward, and is a neurological test ordinarily used for stroke, brain tumor, or brain damage.

When I scraped the bottom of John Patterson's right foot, both legs rose from the bed, bent at the knees, until both thighs were up against his belly and chest.

I stepped back in complete surprise. I had never seen a reaction like that before, nor had I ever heard of one described such as that.

"Did you move your legs deliberately like that, John, or did they move by themselves?"

"I didn't move them, Doctor, honest. They moved like that by themselves."

"Well, let's do it again, John, and see if we get the same result. But we'll wait a moment so that I won't catch you in a refractory period when I perform this test again."

A few minutes later, I repeated the maneuver and got the same astounding result.

"Are you sure you're not moving your legs deliberately, John?" I said again.

"I can't move my legs, Doctor. Please believe me. They go up like that by themselves."

"Well, I have to tell you I've never seen anything like that in my entire life, John. And I don't think many other physicians have seen that type of reflex, either. Is that why the other physicians think you can walk because your legs move like that?"

"They never did that test on me, Doctor. They think I'm a malingerer because they couldn't find anything on the x-rays and on the physical examination."

"I think that what we're seeing is the first clue to what is going on in your body, John. Now you relax while I go downstairs and dig out your x-rays. Then I'm going to the medical library to see if any other physicians have ever seen a reflex like yours and have written about it. I'll be back but it may take a few hours."

John Patterson took my hand as I turned to leave and kissed it again.

"Now John," I said. "You're going to make me feel like the Pope. Then I'll be spoiled and expect the same treatment from everybody."

John was crying openly now.

"You just wait, John," I said, touching his cheek and feeling the warm tears on his skin. "I'll be back as soon as I complete my detective work."

In the Radiology Department, I put John Patterson's x-rays on the view box and tried to act like a radiologist. I knew that the typical radiologist spent only ten seconds on a chest film and only a few seconds more on a spine film. Therefore, I had to make up for my inexperience with careful study. I examined the outline of every vertebra in his thoracic and lumbosacral spine repeatedly. They all appeared normal, but as I stepped back and viewed the films from a distance of three feet, there seemed to be a hazy outline of an irregular mass adjacent to the tenth-to-twelfth thoracic vertebrae. I looked more closely. The hazy mass seemed to disappear. Was I reading something in the film that wasn't there? I turned to the report. It stated simply that there was no abnormality of the thoracic and lumbosacral spine. I looked at the film once more. I again saw the hazy outline of a mass. And it wouldn't go away with repeated viewing. Oh well, I thought to myself, if I make a complete ass of myself at Grand Rounds, I can always defend myself by saying, "What do you expect from an intern with no training in radiology?"

I retreated to the library, taking the x-rays with me. I wasn't going to allow them to be "accidentally" lost. This had happened to misinterpreted x-rays before.

I examined every book and every article in the library that had anything to do with neurology and found nothing to explain the phenomenon I elicited from John Patterson. I was disappointed. After two hours, I was about to give up when I noticed in the corner of the library near the entrance, a shelf loaded with old books. A sign stated that these books were going to be discarded and the staff physicians could take them if they so desired. The first book I picked up was entitled, "The Neurological Examination." It was published in 1920. I flipped it open to a discussion of the Babinski reflex and there was my answer. The reflex was named after a physician in Paris, Josef Francois Felix Babinski, who first discovered it in 1896. In certain unusual cases, and very infrequently, a massive response will be elicited when performing the Babinski reflex, during which the lower extremities, bent at the knees, will automatically rise until the anterior thighs are up against the belly and chest, indicating a serious involvement of the central nervous system. The spinal cord is an important part of the central nervous system.

I nearly went into a dance as I felt the adrenalin race through my body.

I took the book with me and returned to the ward.

"John," I said. "I believe you. I believe you. I was crazy to have even the slightest doubt. I've got proof now. I'll have the nurse get you ready for a spinal tap."

Mrs. Christopher was on duty, another one of God's gifts to nursing.

"We're too busy doing meds now, Doctor," she said impatiently. "Schedule it for Monday."

"Are you going to help me or you going to force me to do it by myself?"

She looked at me and saw that I was determined.

"Oh, all right," she said angrily. "But why do you have to do it on your time off? Who is the patient?"

"John Patterson," I said, isolating each word.

"John Patterson!" she screeched. She made a quick maneuver to hold her false teeth in. "Why are you wasting your time on a bum like that? Do you need the practice?"

"Just set it up, please," I said.

The procedure went smoothly. I had the distinct feeling that Mrs. Christopher was hoping I'd screw it up some way. She hovered over us like an old vulture, mad as hell, constantly looking at her watch. The spinal fluid appeared clear. I hooked up the manometer to check the pressure gradients. There was no movement of the fluid level, indicating a block.

"The spinal fluid was clear, Doctor," Mrs. Christopher said, almost happy that I could be barking up the wrong tree. The spinal fluid is frequently cloudy with abnormal conditions. She was exploring with her statement but I didn't bite.

"Yes, it is," I said and let the matter drop. She didn't catch the manometer readings and I wrote a non-specific note in the chart. I wasn't going to let her in on my findings and impression until I was good and ready with all the results.

On Monday, I ordered a series of blood tests on Patterson because nothing had been done on him for a month. By Wednesday I had all the information I needed. There were one hundred lymphocytes in the spinal fluid, which was definitely abnormal. The protein level was also high. I called Tim Murphy, the previous intern, who was now a first-year neurosurgical resident.

"I've been working on John Patterson, Tim," I said.

"You're wasting your time," he said.

"I don't think so, Tim," I said. "Will you come down and take a look at what I've found?"

"OK," he said, "but it'd better be good."

He was down in five minutes and looked over the results I had just entered into the chart.

"Jesus Christ," he said. "This poor son-of-a-bitch is dying with a tumor and we've been calling him a malingerer."

He reexamined Patterson and agreed with my diagnosis. He had never seen a massive withdrawal Babinski reflex like the one Patterson exhibited. He even saw the faint outline of the tumor on the x-ray film just as I had.

"I'll call Dr. Moriarty today and he'll see him in consultation tomorrow and probably schedule him for surgery on Monday. What made you suspicious that he wasn't a malingerer?"

"When I first saw him," I said, "he looked like a dying man pleading for help and I believed him, that's all."

The next day, Thursday, Dr. Moriarty, the chief of neurosurgery, saw Patterson in consultation. He complimented me on the work I had done and scheduled him for surgery on Monday.

The following day, Friday, Dr. George Milton appeared for Grand Rounds at ten in the morning. The second-year medical resident was there, along with the chief resident and the two floor nurses. Two other interns from the other medical floors were also in attendance.

When we came to Patterson's bed, Dr. Milton continued to walk past, even hastening his stride a bit.

"Dr. Milton," I said firmly. "Would you please wait a moment? I have something spectacular to show you regarding a physical finding on Mr. Patterson."

"Doctor." Dr. Milton said impatiently, "I haven't seen anything spectacular since I myself was an intern."

I went over to John Patterson and winked at him. He smiled back and touched my hand. I pulled back the bed covers, exposing his skinny legs, and scraped the bottom of his right foot with the tip of my reflex hammer. Both legs came up in the same unusual manner as they had done before.

I turned around to face all the others, very pleased with myself and ready to take a bow. They all looked bored.

"Well, Doctor, what is it that you want to show us that is so spectacular?" Dr. Milton said.

"I just did," I said. "That is a massive withdrawal Babinski reflex. You'll probably never see another one like that the rest of your lives. That's how rare it is."

7

"You are wrong, Doctor," Dr. Milton said. "You just proved to us that he can really move his legs and should be able to walk."

He turned to go to the next bed and the others began to follow. Mrs. Christopher had a dirty smirk on her face that she could have used as a Halloween mask, but at least her false teeth weren't slipping out.

"Can you give me a few more minutes, Dr. Milton?" I said.

Dr. Milton looked at his watch.

"You know, Doctor, it is getting late and we have many a mile to go before we're done today."

Ah, the good doctor has read Robert Frost, I thought to myself as I remembered the poem "Stopping by the Woods on a Snowy Evening."

"I think you'll find these next things interesting, Dr. Milton," I said. "I reviewed the x-rays on Mr. Patterson and I believe they have been misread."

"How much training have you had in radiology, Doctor?" Dr. Milton said, sarcasm beginning to creep into his voice. There was no doubt in my mind he was becoming hostile.

"Just what the usual medical student gets, Dr. Milton," I said, "which, of course, is not very much."

"And just what do you see on these x-rays that have been misinterpreted by our radiologists, Doctor?"

"I see the faint outline of a tumor adjacent to T-10-11 and 12 on the left."

"Did you review your findings with Dr. Fisher, our radiologist?" Dr. Milton said.

"No, I didn't," I said, "but I have the x-rays here for you to review if you would like to."

I knew that as an internist he didn't know much more about x-rays, either.

"No, I don't believe I'll follow you on this wild-goose chase," he said coldly.

Dr. Milton turned to go.

"There's more, Dr. Milton," I said.

"I believe we've spent enough time on Mr. Patterson already," Dr. Milton said, now getting angrier. "Do you understand me, Doctor?"

"I do understand you, Dr. Milton, but these are Grand Rounds and according to your own written instructions, may I quote: 'The purpose of having Grand Rounds is to bring unusually interesting cases before the entire group so that both the patient and the physician may benefit from the presentation.' I have more to say on Mr. Patterson and I really feel you shouldn't leave until you've heard everything. I promise you it will be rewarding."

"Continue, Doctor, please continue. I can see that you have created a roadblock here. But let me warn you. This is just the beginning of your internship and we will not let you obstruct Grand Rounds like this every week."

"I had Dr. Tim Murphy review the case," I said. "You know that he is now a first-year neurosurgical resident and he agrees with my impression of this case."

"So that's it," Dr. Milton said, his voice louder. "You've managed to convince Dr. Murphy, who first came up with the diagnosis of malingering, to change his mind, Doctor. No doubt Dr. Murphy has made spectacular strides this past week in neurosurgery. But you haven't changed my opinion. Patterson is a malingerer and that's the final word this morning."

It was obvious he didn't plan on listening any more.

The entire group followed him to the next bed.

"Have we got someone to present this next case?" Dr. Milton said politely, in contrast to his previous outburst.

I remained at the foot of John Patterson's bed. Dr. Milton turned around and saw me still standing there.

"Are you coming, Doctor?" Dr. Milton called out. "Or are you glued to the floor?"

"I haven't finished yet, Dr. Milton," I politely called back.

"I'll let you make one more statement to convince me and that will be final," Dr. Milton said.

He stood standing in the middle of the ward with his hands on his hips, the chip on his shoulder balanced precariously, threatening me to knock it off.

"Dr. Moriarty, our Chief of Neurosurgery, has seen Mr. Patterson in consultation and has agreed with my diagnosis. He has written a note in the chart to that effect and has scheduled Mr. Patterson for surgery on Monday."

"Well, goddammit, why didn't you say that in the first place?" Dr. Milton roared.

He turned to leave the ward.

"Rounds are over, gentlemen."

John Patterson grabbed my hand as I started to join the rest of the group.

"Thank you, Doctor," he said.

"No kissing, John," I said, smiling.

There were tears in his eyes, but he was smiling, too.

At surgery the following Monday, Dr. Moriarty found an inoperable malignant tumor compressing the spinal cord at T-10-11-12. Patterson died three months later.

LESSONS TO BE LEARNED

The main problem was the lack of communication that developed between the patient and the physicians in charge. There were two elements that contributed to this sad situation. The most important barrier to communication was the inflexibility of the physicians. When the passive nature of the patient was added to that one facet of the problem, then proper care was totally blocked. Studies have indicated that the more aggressive patient receives better medical care, even though he may be more difficult to handle. Doctors shudder when a patient pulls out a sheet of paper with a long list of complaints. But if the physician takes the time to discuss each item on the list, that patient leaves the office fully satisfied.

John Patterson knew that he couldn't walk but didn't adequately convey his feelings to the physicians. Perhaps it was fear that prevented him from being more aggressive. He knew the other physicians didn't believe him and were angry with him. Instead of becoming more aggressive, he withdrew from the fray and was totally neglected from then on. Could a similar situation develop today? Because of utilization committees, physicians wouldn't be allowed to keep a patient in the hospital for a month without having him under active treatment. A patient like John Patterson would be dumped into a long-term rehabilitation hospital and would continue to be deprived of adequate care unless a nurse or a doctor took a special interest in him.

The worst offense in this case was an inadequate history. The patient had no previous history of malingering nor any other workmen's compensation injury. A diagnosis of conversion hysteria could have been considered but one look at the patient would have thrown out that impression.

PATIENT BEWARE—

The central problem was the stubborn and unyielding nature of the involved physicians. It's so easy to get upset and then angry when the patient doesn't fit into the exact mold we have created for him in our minds. This could have been avoided with a carefully detailed history, including documentation of previous injuries. Then it would have been easier to recognize the fact that the patient had no reason to lie to the physician consciously or subconsciously. What is missing here, too, is a careful follow-up of the patient's problem. John Patterson was dumped and left there unattended. There is no rule in medicine that a proper diagnosis has to be established on the first encounter. At the end of a work-up, we are taught to record our impression of the problem, not necessarily the specific diagnosis. In the early stages of a disease it is frequently impossible to come to a definitive conclusion. A careful follow-up with repetition of essential laboratory and x-ray studies is necessary in all cases if we are to practice high-quality medical care. Subsequent careful observation will lead to the correct diagnosis if the initial evidence is sparse or is wrongly interpreted.

Careful follow-up was totally absent in this case. Instead, the physicians became angry with the patient. They were even intolerant of any other physician who was willing to listen to the patient and reexamine him. This became an insurmountable barrier for both the patient and his original physicians.

The initial x-rays were misread. If the x-rays had been repeated in a reasonable length of time, this mistake would have been corrected. One important physical sign, the massive withdrawal effect that is so rare that most physicians never see it, was misinterpreted. The automatic movement of the lower extremities convinced the doctors that the patient could walk. This type of Babinski reflex was a new and unfamiliar reaction to them. Once the physicians suspected malingering, they shut their minds to any further logical reasoning.

The physician must approach each patient with a certain amount of humility, recognizing the fact that just around the corner from his own great and awe-inspiring ego is another physician equally well-trained who is capable of doing just as good a job or perhaps even better. Once a physician assumes he is infallible and that his care is the best available, disaster looms ahead.

You must remember that even malingerers and neurotic individuals eventually die of various diseases and degenerative conditions. This type of patient forces the physician to work harder to arrive at the correct diagnosis because the patient has frequently strewn the path with many misleading signs and symptoms. However, frustration should not lead to anger. With diligence and a complete and thorough work-up, all these obstacles can be overcome.

Chapter Two

A Grand Old Man

I do not like thee, Dr. Fell,
The reason why I cannot tell,
But this I know and know full well,
I do not like thee, Dr. Fell.
                    Children's Nursery Rhyme

I arrived at the hospital in San Francisco at 7:30 a.m. sharp, one-half hour early for my month of Ob/Gyn training. There were no facilities for this type of training at our base hospital so arrangements were made to take that training at another hospital across town.

As I opened the front door, I heard my name being paged. I grabbed the nearest phone at the information desk in the lobby.

"Where have you been?" a nurse sputtered into the phone. "Dr. Stone is all upset and is ranting and raving like a maniac. You're supposed to do a history and physical on a patient of his who is scheduled for surgery at 8:00 a.m. Please hurry or all our heads will roll."

I looked at my watch. It was 7:35 a.m. I didn't even know they were aware of my name and they were already paging me.

I performed a quick history and physical on Dr. Stone's patient. We were not allowed to do pelvic examinations on these private patients, which made the diagnosis more difficult to determine. She complained of a lump in her right groin. It was hard as a rock to palpation, painless, and immovable, all signs of a cancer that had spread to her groin. She was only thirty-five years old. I wrote her up in the chart quickly with "Metastatic Carcinoma to the Right Groin" as my diagnosis. Then with the help of the nurses we rushed her and the chart to the operating room where Dr. Ralph Stone was stomping around like a wild animal even though we had the patient there in plenty of time.

I heard my name being paged again. It was the chief resident.

"Where have you been?" he said. "You were supposed to report here at eight o'clock."

I looked at my watch. It was 8:05 a.m. I explained to him what had happened.

"Come on up to the delivery-room suite on the third floor north wing," he said. "We're just starting a patient on Pit."

An intravenous drip of Pitocin was used to initiate labor in pregnant women at or around their due dates. By the time I got to the floor, the chief resident and the second-year resident had already started the i.v. drip.

"We're going for coffee," the chief resident said. "I think she'll be slow starting her labor. We'll be back in about twenty or thirty minutes. Keep an eye on her while we're gone."

They took off down the hall along with the nurses.

I looked at my watch. It was 8:10 a.m. It was just forty minutes ago that I had entered this hospital, a complete stranger, only identified as a physician by the stethoscope in my pocket and the fact that I was dressed like an intern. I had already performed a complete history and physical on a young woman dying from cancer and was now initiating labor in a pregnant woman I had never met before. Fortunately, I had had considerable training in obstetrics while I was at Rochester in my fourth year of medical school. Both the intern and the resident had been sick during my stint so I delivered babies like an old pro.

I casually waltzed into the patient's room.

"Well, Mrs. Johnson," I said cheerily. "How are you doing?"

"The baby is coming," she said.

"It can't be," I said. "The chief resident said you'd be a slow starter and you've had the i.v. drip going only ten minutes."

"Doctor," Mrs. Johnson said firmly, in between grunts, "this is my third baby and when I tell you the baby's coming, *the baby is coming.*"

"Let me take a peak," I said, hoping she was wrong.

15

I lifted the sheet, placed my hand on her belly, and took a quick look. She was having a massive contraction and I could see a bit of the baby's head.

"You're right, Mrs. Johnson," I said calmly.

I clamped off the i.v. Pit, whisked her onto a stretcher that was outside her room and rushed her into the delivery room, which was only two doors down. There were no nurses around. They had gone for coffee with the residents. Great deal, I thought. What the hell did these people do before I got to this hospital?

The delivery went smoothly and within five minutes, I had a screeching, squirming, slippery baby in my hands. I tied off and cut the cord and then placed the baby in the incubator. I massaged Mrs. Johnson's belly and the placenta came out almost immediately. The uterus was tight and firm.

Five minutes later, I was wheeling both the mother and the baby down the hall to maternity and the newborn nursery where two surprised nurses greeted me.

"Where's everybody and who are you?" one of them said.

"They're down having coffee," I said. "I'm the janitor."

I went back to the delivery room and completed my notes. I picked up the newspaper on the desk and leaned back, feeling very satisfied with myself. I looked at my watch. The whole affair had taken only fifteen minutes.

I was sitting there very comfortably when the chief resident and the second-year resident returned from their coffee break.

"How is Mrs. Johnson?" the chief resident asked.

"Fine," I said, looking up briefly from the paper. I yawned and stretched out my arms.

The two residents sauntered up the hall to Mrs. Johnson's room.

They ran back in a panic.

"What did you do with Mrs. Johnson?" the chief resident said. His face was red and he appeared very excited.

"I stopped her Pit," I said.

"You stopped her Pit!"

His eyes nearly fell out of his head.

"Who gave you the authority to do that?" he yelled out, his arms waving wildly.

"You did," I said. "You said 'keep an eye on her.' In my book, that means do what is necessary."

"Well, where the hell is she?"

"I delivered her baby and I brought him to the newborn nursery. Mrs. Johnson is now in maternity and she is having a snack right at this moment. Both are doing very well."

"You're kidding," the chief resident said.

"I'm not kidding," I said. "And if you two bastards ever do that to me again, I promise you, I'll castrate both of you."

They ran down to the maternity ward and the newborn nursery to verify what I had told them.

When they came back, the chief resident was smiling.

"Mrs. Johnson is so happy that we placed her in the hands of such a capable doctor," he said.

"You guys placed her in the hands of a total stranger," I said. "You were lucky this time."

The next day was pleasant and quiet. I finally had time to breathe. I went up to the surgical floor and took out the chart on that first patient I had seen so hurriedly for Dr. Stone the previous day. My history and physical had big red slashes across the notes. In the margins, again in red ink, were several caustic comments: "You idiot! Are you a physician or a garbage collector? Don't you know the difference between a cyst of the canal of Nuck and cancer? How dare you write a history and physical like this rot on a patient of mine!"

As I read Dr. Stone's comments, I felt my face getting hot. I looked up and saw the nurses standing there observing my reaction.

"Well," I said. "I certainly made an impression on Dr. Stone, didn't I? The first day on the job, too. Who is that little son-of-a-bitch, anyway?"

"Dr. Stone is Professor Emeritus of Ob/Gyn at this hospital. He was Chief of Surgery for the last twenty years. And he loves to pick on interns."

"I can see that," I said. "Who wants to take a bet that my diagnosis is right and the old fart is wrong?"

One of the younger nurses stepped forward.

"I'll bet that you're right, Doctor," she said.

"I'll let you know as soon as I get the path report," I said. "Furthermore, I never heard of any anatomical lesion like a cyst of the canal of Nuck, and I never heard of the canal of Nuck, either."

Two days later, I was assigned another one of Dr. Stone's patients, a woman of thirty with a mass in her lower abdomen.

"What is Dr. Stone planning to do with you?" I asked, sitting on the edge of the bed.

She appeared frightened and looked away from me quickly. Her hands were clasped tightly against her abdomen as if in defense against the surgery that was scheduled for the next day.

"I really don't know," she said. "All I know is that he has me scheduled for an exploratory to find out what that lump is in the lower part of my abdomen."

"Did Dr. Stone discuss any of the possible diagnoses regarding that lump so that you could give the hospital an 'informed consent' to surgery?"

She quickly looked away again.

"He said that's what the exploratory is for—to find out what that lump is. I just hope it isn't cancer. He didn't explain anything more than that."

She spoke rapidly in a high-pitched voice, the words tumbling out barely formed.

"Has he done a pregnancy test on you?" I asked quietly. I spoke slowly and softly, trying to calm her down by the tone of my voice.

"No," she said. "Dr. Stone said that was unnecessary because he was positive I wasn't pregnant."

Again she looked away quickly.

"Are you having regular periods?"

"No," she said. "I have an underactive thyroid so I'm totally irregular. And to make it worse, I frequently forget to take my thyroid pills."

"When was your last period?"

She looked out the window.

"About two months ago, I think. I really can't remember. My husband and I have been married for 12 years and I've never been pregnant and never did anything to prevent pregnancy, so I stopped keeping track of my periods long ago."

She finally turned to look at me. Her eyes were unfriendly.

"Do we have to go over all of this again? I gave Dr. Stone's nurse the entire history in his office."

"My job," I said, "is to record the history and physical examination for the hospital records. It will only take a few more minutes."

I had to be very careful because I knew I was deep in treacherous waters. This was a private hospital and I knew that some surgical procedures were performed without proper documentation. Furthermore, as I mentioned before, we were not allowed to do pelvic examinations on these private patients, but we were permitted to do rectal exams. Palpating a six-week intrauterine pregnancy through the rectum would be more difficult and I had to be absolutely sure of my findings for the old tyrant, Dr. Stone.

I finished the history and physical and retreated to the nurse's station to write my notes. Mrs. Mildred O'Brien, the head nurse, was there.

"I suppose I'll see a lot of red slash marks on my notes tomorrow," I said, "but I have to put down what I believe, including the fact that a pregnancy test wasn't done."

"What's your diagnosis, Doctor?" Mrs. O'Brien asked.

"Intrauterine Pregnancy, three months gestation," I answered.

"Were you able to palpate the uterus?"

Another nurse had been in attendance during the examination.

"Not as well as doing a pelvic exam," I said.

"So what do you base your diagnosis on, Doctor?" Mrs. O'Brien said, giving me the wise-old-nurse look as a warning.

"On a very carefully taken history," I said, "and, of course, the rectal exam we're stupidly restricted to."

"Tomorrow we'll give you a decent burial with full military honors, Doctor," she said, clicking her tongue and wagging her head. "You can count on it, and you're so young, too."

"I survived WWII, the Wehrmacht, the Nazi SS troops and I'll survive Dr. Stone, too," I said. "He's just an old dog with a big growl masquerading as a lion."

"We'll see," she said. "We'll see."

The next day at surgery, Dr. Stone made a vertical incision and quickly opened up the patient's abdomen. There before our eyes was a pregnant uterus, enlarged about three months, typically cyanotic, with engorged veins, a textbook picture.

"Well, what do you think, Doctor?" Dr. Stone asked the resident.

The resident was hesitant.

"Well, sir...," he said slowly.

"Come on, come on," the old fart said. "We haven't got all day."

"I believe it's an intrauterine pregnancy, sir."

"It's right under your nose and you still can't give me the correct diagnosis. What kind of doctors are we training today? How about you, Doctor? You're obviously an expert. What is your considered opinion?"

He looked straight at me.

"I wrote the history and physical yesterday, Dr. Stone, and my impression then was 'Intrauterine Pregnancy, three months gestation,' and I believe what we are seeing now confirms the diagnosis."

"I suppose there's no room for argument," Dr. Stone said.

"No," I said. "I don't believe so."

"Smart asses," Dr. Stone said, sarcastically. "Is George Foster outside? I know that he was finishing up a case when we started. Ask him if he would be so kind as to step in here for a moment to give us the benefit of his opinion."

What kind of game is this old son-of-a-bitch playing, I thought to myself.

The circulating nurse stepped out into the hallway and a minute later, Dr. Foster came in and took a quick look.

"That's a three-month intrauterine pregnancy, Ralph. Why did you open her up?"

Dr. Foster left before Dr. Stone could give him an answer.

"Well, we shall soon see," Dr. Stone said.

My eyes flicked to the clock on the wall. It took sixty seconds for Dr. Stone to slice the uterus out of the patient's body, leaving the stump of the cervical neck inside, an inexcusable procedure since he left in the part that could become cancerous in the future.

Balancing the uterus on the patient's belly, Dr. Stone made one quick incision revealing its contents, a tiny, fully formed fetus.

"Well, I guess you gentlemen were right after all," Dr. Stone said abruptly. "Close up."

He turned and left the room.

"Why, that son-of-a-bitch should be in jail," I said. "Why do they let him operate?"

"Sh-h-h," the resident said. "If he heard you he could bust you out of medicine."

"And we could bust him in court," I said.

"Busting an old man is no big thing," he said. "But busting a good young physician at the beginning of his career would be a disaster."

We closed without saying another word.

Three weeks later, while going through a batch of pathology reports, I came across the final report on the first patient I had seen in this hospital. That was the patient I had diagnosed as "Metastatic Carcinoma to the right groin"; the history and physical that Dr. Stone had slashed with his red pen; the one where he had written all those vile remarks. The report confirmed my initial impression. I knew it would. I made copies of the report and gave one to each of the nurses on the surgical floor.

The head nurse said, "We know he's bad but he has contributed so much to the hospital, he's like God here."

"I've only got one more week at this hospital so I can't help you to do what you all know has to be done. He's not God. He's the devil."

My final week was uneventful. I never saw Dr. Stone again. I never found out if the staff was able to force him to retire before he did more harm.

LESSONS TO BE LEARNED

Dr. Stone is the type of physician who is obviously dangerous. He treads his path with a heavy foot and a total disregard for the rest of humanity. No humility exists in this individual. His ego is like a voracious monster within him that has to be fed constantly. Was he like this all his life or did he develop these traits as he became an old man, resentful of the young doctors around him? His technical ability as a surgeon could not excuse this terrible defect in his personality. How much pleasure should a mature physician derive out of ripping an intern to shreds on a questionable diagnosis when no harm is done to the patient? He was supposed to teach, not tear to bits. The true nature of this man was revealed when the pathology report was finally issued and he didn't have the courage to discuss it with the intern.

Could a patient really have a two-way conversation with such a physician? Absolutely not. A patient wouldn't dare to ask him any questions.

With an incomplete work-up and a lack of concern for her welfare, this same surgeon took a pregnant woman to surgery with his mind already made up as to what he planned to do. Did he take his own history from the patient? No! His office nurse recorded it.

I have to admit that perhaps the patient did play a part in steering the surgeon towards a hysterectomy instead of accepting a normal pregnancy. She over-emphasized the doctor's opinion that this was definitely not a pregnancy. She seemed unconcerned that a pregnancy test hadn't been done. Was she hiding something? She just may have had complete faith in her surgeon. If he said she wasn't pregnant, then she wasn't pregnant.

I had a feeling at the time that she wouldn't have minded a

hysterectomy even if she had known she was pregnant. This whole affair could have been prearranged.

But if so, the actions of the surgeon are even more damning. He was going to excise that mass no matter what the consequences. As for asking others who were in attendance at his surgical crimes for their opinions, that was initially perplexing to me. Perhaps he did this to continue the charade and also to demonstrate exactly how little he regarded the thoughts of his colleagues. Nobody in that operating room that day dared to come to the rescue of the patient.

As for the residents abdicating their duties to a total stranger who happened to be garbed in the whites of an intern, with no senior nurse, or for that matter, any nurse on the floor, this was sheer folly. When I think back to that moment, I am still appalled.

I have to admit one thing, however. It turned out to be excellent training and I learned a lot. But that doesn't mean that patients should be exposed to this type of care.

Chapter Three

A Definite Cure

Gregory Hamilton woke up with a start. He saw the shadows on the wall. They seemed to move and gradually rearrange themselves until he saw the distinct outline of his three-year-old son lying dead beneath the dash, crumpled like a discarded rag doll, his neck twisted at an odd angle. Gregory Hamilton didn't know what had hit him, but the impact had thrown his son forward with tremendous force.

He started to cry again. His depression came over him like a monstrous wave, hurling him forward on its crest with an increasing rush and then sucking him under, deeper and deeper.

No, not again, he thought to himself. God, not again.

He reached for the phone and accidentally knocked it to the floor. He finally managed to switch on the light and dial the number.

"Dr. West," he said as soon as the receiver was lifted. "Can you come over? I'm bad tonight."

"I'll be right over," Dr. Marilyn West said quickly. "It will take just a few minutes."

"Hurry, please," Gregory Hamilton said. "I can't stand it. I don't know what I'll do if this doesn't stop."

It only took her five minutes to reach his room from the residents' quarters. She pulled a chair over to his bed and took his hand. His whole body was trembling and he was sobbing.

With his other hand he pulled the covers over his head.

She sat there holding his hand until he gradually stopped crying and shaking. She hadn't said one word since she had entered the room.

But now she began to talk to him quietly.

"Will you be all right now, Gregory?" she said.

"Yes," he said from beneath the covers, his voice muffled.

"Are you sure, Gregory? I can stay longer if you want me to."

"No, I'm all right now," he said. "I just saw those shadows on the wall again, Doctor. I thought they were gone for good."

"They soon will be, Gregory," she said. "It won't be long now, I promise you."

"Do you still think you can help me without using pills? Sometimes I feel so bad I feel like I need some kind of medication."

It was eleven months since she had taken over his case. Dr. Percy Carleton, the Chief of Psychiatry had assigned Gregory Hamilton to her as an interesting experiment. He wanted to see if she could restore this man to his previous dynamic existence during her last year of residency without the use of medication.

"Just talk, talk, talk, and nothing more," Dr. Carleton had said.

"Nothing more?" she said.

"Well, just one thing more," he said. "You have to be available when he needs you. You won't be able to abandon him even for short periods of time, unless you have prepared him properly to be able to exist without you being near."

"That's like being shackled to him," Dr. West said.

"And that's exactly what you have to avoid if you are to be successful in this experiment. You have to make him feel totally independent by the time your residency ends. You have exactly one year."

Gregory Hamilton had been found by the police at the scene of the automobile accident sitting in his car crying, holding the body of his dead son in his lap, uttering an endless stream of unintelligible sounds, rocking back and forth, unable to answer the simplest questions or even to identify himself.

He had picked up his son at his mother-in-law's house just twenty minutes before the fatal crash. One year before that he had been in a similar crash that had killed his wife.

Gregory Hamilton had been a successful trial lawyer until the moment of his son's death. He had mourned his wife but had been able to control his grief by working. He was a mixture of Gregory Peck, Gary Cooper, and Laurence Olivier. When he spoke to the jury, his words were like verbal paintings splashed with an amazing intensity of color, propelled by a beautiful voice that mesmerized the twelve individuals sitting in front of him. He was able to project himself in any role he felt obligated to assume, from aristocrat to common man, and so convincingly that the jury accepted his sincerity without the faintest doubt. His colleagues wilted at the thought of facing him in court.

But on the day of his son's death, he became a useless sack of protoplasm, crying constantly and uttering an endless stream of gibberish, rocking back and forth, staring straight ahead and seeing nothing.

That was the way Dr. West found him the first day she met him. It was two weeks after the accident. She entered the room and sat down beside him, taking his right hand with her two hands. She said nothing. She would sit with him an hour at a time, just holding his hand. At first, the sounds from his mouth were a wild torrent, as if each sound bumped and smashed against one another in a mad attempt to escape from his throat. Gradually, they slowed down, like a river reaching a placid pool. Finally there was silence. Then the rocking stopped. Two weeks later, he turned towards her as she entered his room and saw her for the first time.

"Who are you?" he said. "Are you my mother?"

"No," she said. "I'm your doctor."

From then on they began to talk. They discussed everything that happened to come into his mind. If he awoke in the middle of the night and felt like talking, she'd be there in five minutes. Every possible subject was debated and argued except one and that was the death of his son.

One day he looked directly at her.

"Do you ever hate God?" he said.

"Yes, every day," she said. "Why do you ask."

"Well, I wish I could believe there is a God just so I could hate him. Does that make any sense to you?"

"Yes," she said. "I can understand that."

Until that point, she had been a virtual prisoner for three solid months. But from then on he was able to tolerate her absence on her days off. He grilled her when she returned as though she had committed a crime.

"Where did you go and what did you do?" he'd ask impatiently.

"Oh, I had such a wonderful time," she said, smiling and waving her hand at him. "I bought a pair of new hiking shoes and a new raincoat. Wasn't that exciting?"

"What else did you do?" he asked, ignoring her teasing.

"I bought three apples to eat at night when I get hungry and then I read about 20 pages of 'A Farewell to Arms' by Ernest Hemingway."

"Then what?"

"Then I fell asleep," she said.

"That's all? Nothing else?"

"That's all. Just another exciting day in the adventures of Dr. Marilyn West, psychiatrist."

They both laughed.

Six months went by and the Chief of Psychiatry warned her that she'd have to start cutting the umbilical cord.

"Yes, I know. He's about ready," she said.

One day when she entered his room, he turned around and looked at her in a different way.

"Are you ready to talk about it?" she said.

"About what?" he said, already dreading what she was going to say.

"About your son's death," she said.

"What's there to talk about?" he said. "He's dead. I killed him. That's the entire story, isn't it?"

"No, it isn't," she said. "I read the accident report. If I remember correctly, it stated that a drunk crossed the median and struck your car head-on."

"Well, I didn't read the accident report," he said, "but the result is the same, isn't it?"

"If you want to continue living here on the top floor of the psychiatric wing of the hospital, feeling that your life ended that day, I suppose you can. If you want to use your son's death as a way to avoid resuming your previous existence, you certainly have the money to accomplish that end. If you feel that the rest of your life should be spent mourning a dead child, a really useless existence, that's your privilege."

"You didn't lose a son," he said.

"That's true," she said. "I understand that you'll never stop grieving. I never asked you to do that. But the human mind is a wonderful thing and there is a place in it to erect that monument to your son without placing it in front of you like an insurmountable barrier. Let it instead be a source of power that grows within you, a force that prevents you from standing in one place, a force that constantly propels you forward to do all the good things that you are capable of doing, for your own satisfaction and for the good of others."

"You forgot to add, 'Let's get one for the Gipper,'" he said, smiling weakly.

She smiled back.

There were more discussions as time went on. He entered into the dialogues with more enthusiasm, and his entire being took on a glow that he thought had been lost forever. And he was proud of the fact that during his entire hospitalization, he hadn't taken any medication. His bridge to a healthy existence was built by two extended hands and the warmth of the human voice. He was determined more than ever not to be addicted to any medication.

I started my psychiatric training at the end of my fourth year of medical school. That's when I met Dr. West. She was preparing to present Gregory Hamilton at Grand Rounds on the day he was to be discharged. For doctor and patient, this was their glorious moment. This was also the last day of her psychiatric residency at Rochester. She was leaving for San Francisco that same day to join a large psychiatric group there.

It was really a joyous day. The happiness emanating from Dr. Marilyn West and Gregory Hamilton seemed to envelop all the students and attending physicians who were there. It was spring, too, of course, when the entire northern hemisphere was charged with a new vigor and rebirth, and the air smelled fresh and clean. Everybody was happy.

At the end of the presentation, we all stood up and clapped and clapped and clapped. Someone even yelled out, "Bravo!" It was an astounding reaffirmation of life. We were all caught up in it. The force that Dr. West ignited in Gregory Hamilton spread spontaneously. It was irresistible. I saw Dr. Percy Carleton beaming with pride. The experiment had worked.

"Now, that's a definite cure and total rehabilitation if I ever saw one," he said to another staff physician who was standing next to him.

One hour later Gregory Hamilton was discharged from the hospital, a cured and rehabilitated individual. He was still smiling.

That night, he was in his own bed, the first time in one year. He was sleeping peacefully, totally relaxed. He awoke with a start. He turned and saw the shadows on the wall. They were faint and constantly rearranging themselves in various indistinct patterns. He looked at them for a long time. They formed and reformed in an endless turmoil, as if moved by some strange force. They remained faint and indistinct. When they didn't emerge in the shape of his son, he turned away, feeling better. Now perhaps he could finally sleep again.

But he lay there in the dark, wide awake, listening to his own breathing and the beating of his heart. Then he began to hear another sound, as if from a great distance, a soft wailing, softer than the beat of his heart, like the faint sound of the wind. It seemed to be coming from behind him.

He turned back and looked at the wall again. The shadows were still moving and rearranging themselves in a constant flow of indistinct patterns. He felt reassured but the sound disturbed him. He thought that he had heard it somewhere before. It seemed to be coming from the wall. It was somehow related to the motion of the shadows, louder as the shadows moved quickly, and softer as their turmoil lessened.

He turned away again, hoping that the sounds would disappear if he stopped looking at the wall. It was useless. He finally rolled over to watch and as he did, the shadows began to gradually rearrange themselves into the distinct outline of his three-year-old son as he plunged forward in slow motion to his death. The sounds were clear now, too. They were the sounds of his son crying as he was thrown forward. He didn't remember hearing them before.

The motion was agonizingly slow, as if his brain had recorded the entire crash and was now projecting it on the wall in slow motion, advancing one frame at a time.

Then it was finally the last frame, punishing him with its brilliance, its intense colors frozen on the wall, his son lying dead beneath the dash, crumpled like a discarded rag doll with his neck twisted at an odd angle.

He turned away and reached for the phone, knocking it to the floor with a loud clattering noise that reverberated throughout the room. He sat up and turned on the light, his head down, afraid to look at the wall. It was quiet now and he sat there for a long time, head down, listening to his heart pound.

He finally looked up. With the light on, the shadows were gone. But he saw the distinct outline of his dead son on the wall. It looked as if it had been painted there.

"No," he said softly.

He didn't cry. He got up slowly, walked to the wall, and touched his son's image there.

He then went down the stairs to the basement and hanged himself.

LESSONS TO BE LEARNED

This unfortunate individual could have been saved. The resident physician underestimated the severity of the patient's depression and overestimated the "cure." Furthermore, just what the physician attempted to prevent, that is a total dependence of the patient on the doctor, occurred and the physician didn't recognize the deception the patient was acting out. Even though the process of weaning the patient had been deliberately started, the patient subconsciously, in an attempt to please the doctor, acted out the process as if it had been thoroughly successful. In psychiatric practice this is not unusual. In general medicine we have other parameters to guide us as the patient improves, such as the blood count, the temperature, etc., but in psychiatry a clever patient can consciously or subconsciously mislead his physician more easily.

In some cases, as in this, a severe depression can have all the appearances of an acute psychotic break with many of the diagnostic features of schizophrenia.

In the present situation we can't expect a severely ill patient like Gregory Hamilton to be able to decide whether he is in the hands of a capable physician. But we can expect a psychiatrist with more experience than a resident physician to be able to discern whether the patient who appears to have made astounding progress has really done so or is merely playing the game of deception, consciously or subconsciously.

It was up to Dr. Percy Carleton, the chief of the department, who had given Dr. West this experiment, to participate more actively in the treatment and to teach the resident physicians a certain degree of wariness since dependence is one of the complications of such a protocol. Dr. Carleton did no follow-up on his own, probably in deference to Dr. West. This situation occurs frequently in academic centers where the resident staff is left to do what they feel is necessary and then learn by their own mistakes. Unfortunately, the mistakes that do occur may be disastrous.

Chapter Four

A Benign Cyst

"*M*arvelous Marv" Templer looked up.

"Is the team ready?" he said through his surgical mask.

"The team is ready and raring to go," the anesthesiologist said.

With one quick motion, "Marvelous Marv" made an incision in the upper outer quadrant of the left breast and revealed the cyst that was palpated as a small ten millimeter mass three days before in my office.

Mrs. Mildred Morton had feared the worst when she first felt the lump. She had come to the office that same day. I had a full schedule but I didn't have the heart to make her wait three days for the first available appointment, while the fear of cancer grew wildly inside her. On physical examination, the mass was slightly tender, but freely movable. A stat mammogram was read as a simple cyst.

She chose Dr. Templer for her surgery. He was the showman of the surgical staff, but capable, and everybody liked him.

With another quick motion, the cyst was in the palm of his gloved hand.

"Now this, gentlemen, is a simple, benign cyst of the breast. Please note its characteristics. It is relatively soft to palpation, slightly tender to the patient, and freely movable, in contrast to cancer, which is usually hard, painless, irregular and immovable."

He handed the specimen to the surgical nurse who deposited it in a specimen bottle filled with a clear solution.

"I'm so positive this is nothing more than a simple benign cyst, we won't waste time by doing a frozen section for cancer. There's no reason to prolong the anesthesia."

He inserted three quick sutures to close the incision.

"This will not even leave a dimple in her breast. I'm sure Mrs. Morton will be pleased about that. Finish up, gentlemen. A gall bladder full of rocks is waiting for me in the next room. Thank you for this pleasant interlude."

Mrs. Morton went home that afternoon, very happy with the news that she didn't have cancer and would not require any further surgery.

Unfortunately, the pathologist disagreed with "Marvelous Marv." The cyst was cancerous. It was my unfortunate task to impart this information to Mrs. Morton and cut short her brief period of joy.

Luckily, we had caught her cancer early. A slightly wider excision was all that was necessary to solve her problem.

She was readmitted a few days later, underwent her definitive surgery, and was discharged in excellent condition the next day. This time it did leave a dimple, but Mrs. Morton was still pleased with the result.

LESSONS TO BE LEARNED

There is one simple lesson here. Even when a breast lump is excised and lies in the palm of your hand, it's frequently impossible to fathom its true nature. Therefore, when the lump is still inside the patient, the physician mustn't procrastinate. It must be taken out. But the full protocol should be followed: surgery plus an immediate frozen section to prove whether the mass is malignant or benign. You won't get any hurrahs shouted from the hilltops for delaying surgery. The fastest growing malpractice cases today are all related to the delayed cancer diagnosis.

One of the patients I've seen recently had been "watched" with a mammogram every three months for a total of nine months for a mildly suspicious lesion in the breast before it was finally excised and proved to be malignant. She was terribly upset, naturally, and was determined to sue. The lesion was still small and caught early (not as early as it could have been), but it took time to convince the patient of this. Of course, the eventual outcome has yet to be determined.

We all know how difficult it is to locate a small suspicious area in the breast and the agony the patient experiences during the process. Occasionally, it is missed entirely on physical examination, only to rear its ugly head at a later date when it might be too late. But procrastination can lead directly to unnecessary suffering by the patient and subsequent costly litigation.

If a physician advises a patient that a period of watchful waiting is indicated because of the "benign" nature of any lump, the patient should insist on a second opinion immediately.

Shortly after I set up practice, I happened to see a fifteen-year-old girl with a high fever. After taking care of that problem, the mother happened to mention she had recently seen a physician because of a lump in her right breast. The doctor had advised careful observation for a period of three months. This frightened the patient but she said nothing. She asked me if she should wait. I examined her and found a fixed, irregular lump in her right breast. Fortunately, there were no palpable nodes. She had immediate surgery and the mass proved to be malignant. She is still alive and well today.

What is careful observation if you don't see a patient for three months? Is that really careful observation or actually neglectful non-observation?

Chapter Five

The Pale Appendix

*I*t was shortly after the last morning service on Sunday that the Reverend Arthur Shipley called me.

"Can you see me this morning, Doctor? I've got the worst stomach ache I've had in my entire life."

I had just gotten home from morning rounds at the hospital and my wife was busy preparing breakfast.

"I should be back in a few minutes," I said to her.

Mr. Shipley was grunting and writhing in pain when I got to his house.

"When did this start, Mr. Shipley?" I said.

"Shortly after the last service, Doctor. My stomach was a little upset since I got up this morning, but the pain didn't start until later."

"I told him to cancel the service," Mrs. Shipley said, "but he refused. I just didn't know what to do."

"Do you feel the pain all over your abdominal area or is it worse in any particular spot, Mr. Shipley?"

"It seems to be generalized, Doctor. There is no particular place that it hurts worse. It's just miserable all over."

His abdomen was soft to palpation. There was no evidence of muscle spasm or rebound pain. Intestinal peristalsis was slightly overactive. His temperature was normal.

"Is it appendicitis, Doctor?" Mr. Shipley said.

"I don't believe so, Mr. Shipley. Your belly is soft and there is

no localized spasm. However, sometimes appendicitis does start this
way, so we'll have to watch you carefully. We don't want you to pull
any surprises on us. At the present time, I feel that you have an acute
gastroenteritis, an inflammation of the intestines. I'm going to give
you an antispasmodic to relieve the pain you're experiencing. Don't
eat or drink anything. I want you to call me in four hours, or sooner if
you think you're getting worse."

"You're sure it's not appendicitis, Doctor?"

"I'm quite sure, Mr. Shipley, although the diagnosis of appendicitis can be difficult to determine early in the disease process. The
classical picture we see is periumbilical pain that gradually migrates
to the right lower quadrant over the subsequent twenty-four hours. Of
course, there are as many variations of that scenario as there are
people. Would you feel better if I sent you to the emergency room for
some blood tests or perhaps even admit you overnight?"

"No," Mr. Shipley said. "I'd rather stay home unless the pain
gets worse."

He appeared very nervous and his wife was clucking over him
like an old hen.

"Would you like me to get another pillow for you, dear?" she
said, straightening out his bed covers.

"Yes, dear," Mr. Shipley said. "I'd like that."

"Try not to worry, Mr. Shipley," I said. "I'll be home all day. If
you need me, I'll be right over."

Mr. Shipley did not last four hours before I got the next call.

"Doctor, my husband is much worse," Mrs. Shipley said over the
phone. "Will you come right over or should I call the ambulance?"

Mrs. Shipley had a new determination in her voice and I got the
distinct impression that she was now in charge of the case and planning the next move.

"I'll be right there, Mrs. Shipley," I said.

Mr. Shipley was still writhing in pain.

"Now let me just feel your belly, for just a brief moment, Mr.
Shipley," I said, trying to calm him down.

"You have to do something right away, Doctor," Mr. Shipley
said. "The pain is unbearable. Call Dr. Wakefield. I just know he'll
have to operate."

His belly was still soft. There was no spasm or rebound pain.

Peristalsis was normal.

"We can't let you stay here and suffer like this, Mr. Shipley. Your belly is just as soft as it was before but I think it would be wise to do a few tests at the hospital to confirm the diagnosis. I'll call Dr. Wakefield and I'm sure he'll meet us at the hospital. I'll take you there myself so that we won't have to waste time waiting for the ambulance."

Dr. Wakefield was the Chief of Surgery. He was a tall, overbearing individual who loved to strut through the hospital, acknowledging the adoration of the masses who lived on the lower level of humanity.

"This is a classical case of acute appendicitis," he said, straightening out to his full godly height after examining Mr. Shipley.

"That's what I thought," Mr. Shipley said, his eyes flicking over to me in admonishment. "When it wasn't getting any better, I just knew it was appendicitis."

"I'll notify the operating room immediately, Mr. Shipley," Dr. Wakefield said. "As soon as I take out that miserable appendix, you'll be all better."

"Thank you, Dr. Wakefield," Mr. Shipley said. "I'm beginning to feel better already."

Again his eyes flicked over to me, as if to say, "I knew it was appendicitis right away but you wouldn't listen."

In the hallway, Dr. Wakefield turned to me.

"You needn't scrub on this one, Doctor. After all, he's a minister and there won't be any fee for you."

"If you don't mind, Dr. Wakefield, I do want to scrub on this case. Mr. Shipley is the minister of a church in town and although I don't belong to his church, I've taken care of him for many years. I certainly wouldn't want him to think that I would desert him when he required surgery. And besides, I want to get a good look at that appendix."

Dr. Wakefield gave me an odd look as he headed for the operating room. I followed him.

It took about thirty minutes to get everything ready. Dr. Wakefield and I were scrubbing when the intern walked in.

"Dr. Wakefield, do you mind if I scrub on this case?" he said. "The white count is only 8000 and I haven't seen any cases of acute appendicitis with normal counts like that."

"By all means, scrub if you like, Doctor. Every case is a learning experience for all of us. After you've been in practice as long as I have, you'll realize how difficult it is at times to make an accurate diagnosis of acute appendicitis. There is no substitute for experience. That is what allows an older surgeon to see beyond simple blood tests and rely on his instinct alone."

Dr. Wakefield made the standard incision in the right lower quadrant. He deftly went through the muscle layers and the peritoneum and then quickly stuck his index finger in the open wound. The appendix was suddenly there for all of us to see. It was pale and healthy. There were no signs of inflammation.

"Now, looking at this appendix," Dr. Wakefield said, his voice assuming an artificially sonorous tone, "you would be tempted to say that this is a perfectly normal appendix. However, I wouldn't be too hasty jumping to that conclusion."

While he was casting his words down like bolts of lightning on us mere mortals, he was busy rubbing the appendix between the first three fingers of his right hand.

"You could be terribly surprised at what the pathologist will say after he views this little miserable vestigial cecal appendage through the microscope."

I looked at the intern. He winked at me. I knew that Dr. Wakefield was not overwhelming him with those fine descriptive phrases.

Two days later, I went down to the pathology lab.

"I had a hard time proving your diagnosis of acute appendicitis, Doctor," the pathologist said somewhat sarcastically, but smiling at the same time. "I gave you the benefit of any question and called it periappendicitis."

"My diagnosis was acute gastroenteritis," I said, "as you already know if you read the chart, Dr. Bowen. The intern agreed with me and scrubbed because he had never seen an acute appendicitis with a normal white count. And if you had seen how Dr. Wakefield rubbed that healthy pale appendix with his fingers, you'd know why you saw so many white cells around the appendix instead of in it, thereby allowing you to call it periappendicitis."

"I know all their tricks, Doctor," the pathologist said. "But I always give the man with the knife the benefit of the doubt."

Mr. Shipley had an uneventful recovery. He went home in three days, extremely happy.

"Here it is only Wednesday," he said, "three days after surgery for appendicitis and I feel great. I feel so good I'm sure I'll be able to hold service this Sunday. Isn't Dr. Wakefield a great surgeon?"

If Mr. Shipley hadn't had surgery, he would have recovered in one or two days and felt even better.

LESSONS TO BE LEARNED

Here is a surgeon who thinks he knows something that nobody else does. We all read the same literature and are exposed to the same statistics. Yes, it's true that in the elderly the same diagnostic criteria do not hold as in the younger age groups. The white count may not respond as quickly or as steeply. But the minister was only 50 years old. I wouldn't call that elderly.

One of the most difficult things for a physician to do is to watch and wait. Today, we are gradually losing sight of the natural course of many diseases because of early intervention. Many of these diseases are naturally overcome by the body's defenses, if the physician doesn't interfere with the body's immune system and prevent it from doing its job. Early intervention can mask this process and the physician then mistakenly attributes the successful outcome to the treatment instead of the body's own healing effect. The human body has everything it needs to heal itself, even against cancer, if it is allowed a chance to do so. It's true that the body can be overwhelmed by the disease process. The treatments of the future will be concerned with unleashing and strengthening the body's own natural defenses.

I once saw an eighty-two year-old woman in my office presenting all the signs and symptoms of acute appendicitis. I called the surgeon of her choice. He told me he would be glad to see her but he knew already that she didn't have appendicitis.

"Ah, a surgeon with clairvoyance," I said. This physician was a good friend of mine.

"Nothing of the sort," he said. "It's so rare for an eighty-two year-old individual to have appendicitis that I'll bet my bottom dollar that I'm right."

"You're going to lose your money," I said. "Your horizons will be expanded today."

It *was* acute appendicitis.

The surgeon in this chapter, however, was playing the game of "Surgeon knows best," and was thoroughly wrong. The charlatan in him caused him to rub the appendix with what he thought was a surreptitious motion. The patient, however, thought he was a genius until I sent him a copy of the path report with a full explanation two weeks later.

But do you think the patient was happy knowing that he didn't require surgery after all? Of course not. He felt guilty about those baleful glances he cast in my direction when the godly surgeon had declared the case to be acute appendicitis.

Dr. Wakefield was an extremely busy surgeon and didn't have to force the issue. His consultant's fee, however, would have been paltry compared to a surgical fee for appendicitis.

Surgeons love to quote statistics like the following: A good surgeon should have 85% of his cases of acute appendicitis supported by microscopic pathological findings. If he is above this average, say 95%, then he is too cautious and waits too long to operate, thereby forcing his patients to suffer the consequences of delayed surgery such as ruptured appendix, peritonitis, and obviously, increased mortality. If his percentage of normal appendices at surgery is above 15%, then he is identified by his colleagues as a surgeon who obviously ignores the basic diagnostic criteria for appendicitis and operates too quickly.

Perhaps Dr. Wakefield in this case was merely attempting to adjust his own statistics. Should we give him the benefit of the doubt like the pathologist did? And knowing how this pathologist adjusted his reports, can we rely on these statistics if this is done in all hospitals?

Chapter Six

A Strange Resemblance

*T*he subject was "Physical Diagnosis by Observation."

"This morning, you are going to depend on your eyes to give you the clue as to the exact diagnosis," Dr. Crane said. "We are going to walk past certain patients in the ward that I will designate beforehand. If you blink or turn away for a split second, the diagnosis may be lost. At the end of each tour, we will stop and discuss our observations and then decide on the diagnosis. Don't be afraid to stare. The first patient is in the last bed on the right in Ward A."

We had been divided into small groups of four students each so we wouldn't be bumping into one another. We followed Dr. Crane down the long aisle between the beds. We must have looked rather odd with our eyes popping out of our heads as we stared at everything we saw. It was eight o'clock in the morning and all the nurses were busy administering treatments and handing out various medications. The lab technicians were flying around drawing blood while other patients were getting into wheelchairs to go down to the x-ray department. Several patients were hooked up to a variety of tubes, i.v. solutions, bladder irrigations, EKG electrodes, and breathing tubes. They were in various stages of a variety of illnesses from mild to serious.

In the last bed on the right, a thin, cadaverous, middle-aged man lay quietly, apparently breathing his last few breaths, as a nurse sat beside him in the hopeless task of trying to feed him. Cereal was dripping down his chin. His cheeks were sunken and his eyes dull. His skin appeared to be a thin, translucent, bloodless membrane, stretched tautly and glued onto his facial bones. His arms and legs were pitifully thin appendages protruding from a completely wasted body. The last time I had seen individuals like that was shortly before World War II ended in May 1945, when our Intelligence and Reconnaissance Platoon liberated a concentration camp in Austria called Gunskirchen.

We stepped out into the hallway and followed Dr. Crane to the conference room.

"Well," he said to us as we sat down.

A few minutes before, as we walked down that aisle, we were all pop-eyed and unblinking, staring carefully at that miserably sick individual in the last bed on the right. But now we were all blinking as rapidly as we could, trying desperately to avoid Dr. Crane's gaze.

"We'll start with our first volunteer, here on my left, and each of you will have a chance to voice your opinion about the diagnosis."

Dr. Crane was pointing at me.

"Well," I said, taking a moment to clear my throat and stalling for time. "I can't give you a definitive diagnosis, but I can tell you that he looks like an inmate from a concentration camp that we liberated just before the war ended in Austria in 1945. He appears to be dying from a wasting disease and the most common example of that today is cancer invading one organ or another."

"Good," Dr. Crane said. "I can see that you've been reading your book on physical diagnosis."

Each man spoke, adding to what the previous person said, but nobody came up with a specific diagnosis.

"I'll give you the first clue," Dr. Crane said. "The patient has an infectious disease."

Again we went around the table. Intractable pneumonia and end-stage syphilis were mentioned as possibilities.

"Why syphilis?" Dr. Crane said.

"Well, it takes ten years to reach your heart, fifteen years to reach your brain, untreated, that is, and it's called the great imitator because it can simulate any disease."

"Good," Dr. Crane said. "Now here is your second clue. Many younger people died of this disease years ago when it was very prevalent. For instance, the name of a famous pianist-composer comes to mind."

"Chopin, tuberculosis," I said.

"Exactly," Dr. Crane said.

"But the patient wasn't coughing," I said. "And furthermore, he isn't isolated and there was no sputum jar on his side table."

"That's right," Dr. Crane said. "His chest x-ray is normal. He has an infectious disease but he himself is relatively not infectious."

"Then how about tuberculosis of the kidneys?" Ray Larkin, another student, said.

"Or what Thomas Wolfe died from, tubercular meningitis," I said.

"All good suggestions," Dr. Crane said, "but we don't have a winner yet."

There was further discussion but nobody in the group was able to come up with the correct diagnosis.

"This man has tubercular peritonitis," Dr. Crane said finally. (The peritoneum is the lining of the abdominal cavity.)

We looked at one another. How could Dr. Crane expect us to identify that exact diagnosis by looking at this patient? That was beyond the realm of reason.

Dr. Crane saw the doubt on our faces.

"I suppose you all doubt that a good clinician could arrive at that diagnosis by just looking at the patient."

We all nodded our heads.

"Well," Dr. Crane said, "I suggest you retreat to the medical library after this session on physical diagnosis and dig up the necessary proof to make you all believers of the apparently impossible. Tomorrow we will take a poll of the believers and I think all of you will be surprised by the results."

I couldn't wait to get back to my room. I had two excellent books on physical diagnosis that I had been poring over for two weeks before this course began. I just couldn't bring myself to believe that a chronic disease process like tubercular peritonitis could make all the patients suffering from that disease develop the same facial appearance.

But I was in for a shock. On a section devoted to facial appearances in various diseases, there was a picture of a patient suffering from tubercular peritonitis who looked exactly like the patient we had just seen.

I'm a believer, I'm a believer, I said to myself, but I still can't believe it. I knew that the people in a concentration camp dying from starvation all begin to look alike, but it was the wasting process that caused the similarity and not any specific disease process. After all, most skulls look alike except to a forensic pathologist. And yet here in my hand was the book on physical diagnosis with a picture of a man with tubercular peritonitis who looked exactly like the patient we had just seen in the hospital. Amazing. I became a believer against my better judgment.

About one month later, I happened to be going through that same ward where we had seen that unusually interesting individual. There was a cluster of people around the last bed on the right. A family had come to the hospital to take their father home after a long illness. I couldn't see too well from the other end of the ward, but a sudden curiosity made me walk towards that bed where we had all been transformed into believers.

It was a happy moment for the entire family. They were all busy packing and getting everything ready to take the patient home, along with his plants and collection of get-well cards. I saw the father, who was our patient of a month ago, as he turned towards me full-face. He looked exactly like he did the month before, except he no longer appeared ill. One of his sons, about twenty, was standing next to him. He looked just like his father. Another son, younger, about sixteen, looked exactly like his brother. A daughter, about fourteen, looked like her two brothers. I looked over at his wife. I half-expected her to look just like her husband, but no, there was no resemblance. I managed to take all this in without forcing my eyes to bug out. I was blinking normally. You can imagine how much I had improved in the art of physical diagnosis in just one short month.

I never saw another case of tubercular peritonitis and I never saw another individual who looked like a member of that family. As the years went by, I managed to develop a healthy skepticism about some of the things I read about in the field of medicine.

LESSONS TO BE LEARNED

There are many interesting things in the field of medicine. Some of them border on the amazing. As an observer, it's easy to come to the wrong conclusions if you view any particular incident superficially. Some of these phenomena have a solid basis in folklore that later can be explained logically and scientifically. Think of the American Indian chewing on the bark of a tree to relieve pain. This was ridiculed by the early settlers and attributed to the ignorance of the savage. Later, it was discovered that the bark contained a chemical that had analgesic (pain-killing) properties. Fifty years ago among the poor and uneducated, children wore cubes of camphor around their necks every summer to prevent polio. I was one of the great mass of poor children who did this. I have no idea where my mother had heard about this medical preventive measure. Only in recent times was it discovered that camphor stimulates the immune system.

In this chapter, our imagination was stretched to the limit. I am still amazed by the sheer coincidence of it all. It would be interesting to take pictures of patients with tubercular peritonitis to see if this resemblance is truly based on fact. With tuberculosis on the rise again in the United States some investigator with a government grant may yet have a chance to do this. However, I'll continue to believe that emaciation was behind it all and not the specific disease. In this particular case, I am sure it was mere family resemblance.

Chapter Seven

Millie

*F*reddie sat in the wooden chair with his feet twisted around the rungs. He kept looking out the window and wringing his hands.

"What are we going to do?" he said. His face was contorted with anguish. There were tears in his eyes.

He spoke to himself, his voice a high wailing sound.

"What are we going to do?" he said again.

His sister Millie didn't look at him. Nothing in her appearance suggested she had heard Freddie. She was frying some bacon and the kitchen was filled with the faint blue smoke rising from the pan. The smell of bacon hung heavy in the air.

She worked with a fierce resolution that was frightening to Freddie. Her eyes smoldered with anger and her lips were tight against her teeth. Her face was covered with a light film of moisture. Freddie knew better than to disturb her when she was in this kind of mood. He sat there twisting his hands and groaning softly, occasionally wiping his nose against his shirt sleeve.

She worked fiercely, as if her life depended on it. She tried to blot out the events of the past two weeks. Each new blow had smashed against her brain without any apparent penetration, but today she suddenly realized it was the end. She couldn't fight back any more. It was just too much for her to bear. Her head began to pound again.

Freddie had come home two hours before with his notice of

termination from the local mill in his pocket. He had handed the slip of pink paper with the neat print to Millie and then sat near the window, his mouth open, drooling, his hands moving constantly, his anguish contorting his face grotesquely. There was an attitude of utter stupidity and helplessness about him.

Millie had looked at the paper and for a moment her brain refused to function. The simple printed words were meaningless. Her whole life seemed to be reflected before her as a frightening void. There was nothing left of her to react to the slip of paper. The bitterness, hatred, and anger that she had lived with the past ten years had consumed the total of her emotions and she felt empty.

She looked at the notice and then let it fall to the table. She felt slightly dizzy as she turned again to the frying pan where the crisp bacon sizzled. With a spatula she lifted the strips carefully and stretched them out on a paper towel. She turned the burner off. She was like a person in a trance, her movements wooden and automatic. But her eyes flashed with their old fierce anger.

There was a sudden movement outside, a stirring of hoofs, a clanging of bells, punctuated by the lowing of cows.

Freddie watched them, the last of his father's dairy herd. There were fifteen of them, healthy, strong, fawn-colored Jerseys. They walked with a deep preoccupation, a profound dullness, chewing continuously, tails flicking, following the farmer up ahead. Now and then one of them quickly turned away with a few fast steps, jumping stiff-legged, and then as quickly, stopping and tearing at the grass edging the road, leaving a fine webbing of saliva in the air. They were clumsy, crude, apathetic creatures. The black wet dirt was lifted into the air by their hoofs.

"That's the last of them, Millie," Freddie said, his voice breaking. "All of Pa's cows gone now."

Millie kept her head down, her face moist and glistening from the heat of the stove, her eyes dangerous with hatred. She pressed the side of her head with her right hand. Her vision blurred as she saw flashing lights and a zig-zag formation.

The sound of the cows gradually faded and everything was quiet. Freddie forgot his anguish for the moment and sat watching a long-legged bug walk up the smooth surface of the window pane.

He looked beyond the bug to the road.

"Oh, I see Mr. Kendall," he said, like a child full of delightful anticipation.

Millie gave no indication she heard Freddie. She placed the bacon on two plates beside thick slices of bread.

"Eat your dinner, Freddie," she said flatly.

"Mr. Kendall's coming here, Millie," Freddie said. Again his voice rang out with delight. He was big and hulking and his movements were gross and clumsy.

He flung open the door and stood there smiling, his eyes shining with expectation.

"Hello, Mr. Kendall," he said joyfully. "Did you bring me anything?"

"Hello, Freddie," Mr. Kendall said. "Hello, Millie. You bet I did, Freddie."

Mr. Kendall reached into his pocket and pulled out a toy rubber dog.

"It squeaks if you squeeze it, Freddie."

Freddie snatched it out of Mr. Kendall's outstretched hand and began to squeeze it furiously. When he heard the squeaking, he broke out with a high-pitched laugh.

Mr. Kendall turned to Millie. His face suddenly looked weary.

"That's the last of the cows, I guess," he said. "Mr. Phillips is getting some fine animals at a bargain price."

Millie nodded.

At the words, Freddie stopped laughing and dropped the toy dog as if he had been bitten. He went back to his chair near the window, his face assuming that look of torment like a cruel mask bolted onto his facial bones. He started wringing his hands and moaning softly.

"It's bad, bad," Mr. Kendall said, "having to sell those fine cows."

Freddie moaned louder.

Mr. Kendall stood in the middle of the room not quite knowing what to do. He was a big, bulky man and his clothes were rather shabby. His scarred hands hung loosely at his sides, still bearing traces of the car grease he couldn't wash off. He was a middle-aged man, the owner of a gas station a mile down the road. He had been a friend of the family a long time, dropping in occasionally for a chat with Millie's father before the latter's unfortunate death. He had watched Millie grow from a chubby girl to a full-hipped, heavy-breasted woman. After his own wife died, his visits became more frequent. His courtship was a peculiarly silent one, Mr. Kendall being content to come and watch Millie out of the corner of his eye. He had never progressed beyond this point because of his own shyness and the wall of silent anger and hatred Millie had built around her.

"And the mill closing down, too," Mr. Kendall said, shaking his head to indicate his profound sorrow.

But inwardly, his sorrow was tempered by a burst of happiness because of the turn of events. Now Millie would have to accept him as a protector, a surrogate father, perhaps even a lover, or husband. He felt a peculiar tingling of his tongue as he thought of this. It would be nice to have a full-hipped young woman like that to share his bed. He would even accept the responsibility of watching over Freddie.

"And I suppose you got your notice from the mill with the rest of them, Freddie," Mr. Kendall said.

Freddie let out a soft, frightened sound from deep in his throat. Tears welled in his eyes. Mr. Kendall threw up his hands and then let them fall to his side.

"Ah," he said with a long sigh. "These are certainly bad times. Who would have thought just a few years ago that this could have happened?"

Millie stood with her back to Mr. Kendall, one hip leaning against the kitchen sink. He loved moments like these when he could watch Millie squarely, observing her heavy-fleshed movements, the tightening of her dress across the side of her full breasts, and watch how her dress revealed the motion of her ample buttocks. His mouth would fill with saliva and he'd catch himself holding his breath. A good strong woman with big hips, he thought, big warm hips.

Millie turned to look at Mr. Kendall, her breasts straining as she breathed quickly. She saw the look on his face and the fear and hatred in her eyes softened for a moment. She knew Mr. Kendall was a good man and that he desired her. She had caught him looking at her many times with an intensity that was all too clear. She liked him, his big clumsy friendliness, but there was something in her that recoiled from him, that took a pleasure in wounding him, that gave her some kind of weird joy to see the pain and loneliness in his eyes, knowing there was another miserable, lost, lonely dependent soul in this world besides herself.

Mr. Kendall turned away. He could feel his face getting hot. He gave a little cough to clear his throat. A good solid woman to drive a man crazy, he thought. When the anger left Millie's face, she was downright pretty. Her lips would relax and reveal their sensual fullness and her blue eyes would be heavy-lidded and inviting.

But these moments were all too brief. When he turned back to her he saw the old fear and anger flash in her eyes. Mr. Kendall found this difficult to understand. He felt confused. It was not just the loss of her farm that made her this way. He thought it was the death of her father that caused the biggest emotional upheaval in her. He wanted to talk to her, to reassure her, to let her know he would help her. But she had erected this terrible barrier and he didn't know how to penetrate it without frightening her more.

"What did the doctor say, Millie?" he finally blurted out.

"The doctor?" Millie said dully, as if she didn't fully understand what Mr. Kendall had said.

"Dr. Morton," Mr. Kendall said.

"Oh yes, Dr. Morton. He said my headaches were due to tension or maybe migraine. He said what I need in the house is a man."

She sounded disgusted.

"What about not being able to sleep?" Mr. Kendall said. "You can't keep going like that, you know."

He sounded worried.

"He said I should get married," Millie said. "Everything would be all better then. We really didn't have more than a few minutes to talk. He was too busy."

"Then you're going to leave after all?" Mr. Kendall asked sadly.

"Yes, tomorrow—Sunday," she said, her voice flat.

"On Sunday too, of all days," he said deploringly. "I tell you today nobody has time for anybody except themselves. The world seems to be full of monsters. People seem to have forgotten how to feel for one another. They appear cold and deadly. But sometimes the monsters we have in our own minds are even worse. They can be more deadly."

Mr. Kendall was surprised to hear himself speak those words. Millie stood looking at the floor, as if she hadn't heard him. She was silent.

"Do you have any idea where you're going?" Mr. Kendall asked.

Again Freddie let out that soft sound of pain from deep in his throat.

"To my cousin outside of Pittsfield," Millie said. "Don't worry, we'll manage. We don't need any help."

She looked at Mr. Kendall briefly and felt a sudden twinge of sorrow as she realized he took her last words as a rebuke.

Mr. Kendall turned to go. He couldn't bear the torture of her flesh any longer.

"I'll drop in again tomorrow," he said, his hand on the door. "If I can help you with anything...?"

Mr. Kendall left quickly. Tomorrow I'll have to say my piece, he thought to himself. She won't have to move. Freddie can help around the garage. She'll make a good wife. His mouth filled with saliva again.

Millie hardly nodded at his receding back. She saw him through the window, slightly bent, walking slowly and deliberately. She felt sorry for him. She thought, why do I treat him so miserably?

She set the table mechanically. The bacon was getting cold. She should have asked Mr. Kendall to stay. He would have liked that.

"Come on, Freddie," she said.

Freddie was playing with the toy dog again and laughing.

He ran to the table and began gulping his food down. His cheeks bulged and saliva drooled from the corner of his mouth.

Millie stood watching him.

Poor Freddie, she thought. What would become of him if they were ever separated? He could just about dress himself and the only job he could do was sweep floors in the mill. But now the mill had closed and they were losing the farm.

She had loved her father deeply, that tall, silent, shy man, stooped and bent, with his rough work-worn hands. How often as a little girl she had fallen asleep on his lap while he rocked away gently in his favorite chair, puffing away on his chewed-up old pipe. She remembered the many times she had awakened during the night frightened by some horrible dream. She'd run to her father's bed and climb up beneath the covers, feeling his big, gentle hands pulling her to him, stroking her hair.

"Dear little girl, how I love you," he'd say softly, hugging her, never thinking what effect their close relationship might have on her in later years.

The good clean smell of his body would be strong in her nostrils, mixed with the smell of tobacco and the faint, sweet odor of hay. The hair on his chest would pinch and tickle.

How simple everything had seemed then.

But now her father was gone and there was only Freddie. Freddie had his father's big-boned body, but where the old man was gentle and agile, Freddie was hulking and clumsy. Every time Millie looked at Freddie she thought of the shy, sensitive old man who had died much too soon ten years ago. How many times had she cried herself to sleep at night. Freddie would hear her and come into her room.

"Why are you crying, Millie?"

"Go to sleep, Freddie," she'd say.

And with his face twisted in sorrow, Freddie would shuffle off to his own room, his mind lost in a cloud of confused images.

The ten years since her father's death had eaten away at Millie's heart like some cunning beast. Slowly her eyes had filled with a wild undirected fear and anger. The young men of the town, first attracted to her, saw this strange anger that flamed about her like some frightening aura, whispered among themselves and finally stayed away. Mr. Kendall was the only one left who still hoped to eventually dissipate that dangerous look in her eyes.

Millie stood looking out the kitchen window listening to Freddie eating noisily behind her. It was getting dark and the rich wet soil around the cow barns seemed black. The main barn loomed against the dimming sky, its base in shadows that merged with the ground.

Empty, she thought. Everything is empty. I am empty, too, an exterior without an interior, a shell. I am an empty room. If only she could feel her father's strong arms holding her again, whispering sweet things into her ear, calling her his "dear sweet child."

As she kept looking out the window, she followed the rise of the ground from the barn to the ridge above. On the highest point of the ridge she saw the slender stone campanile of the church her father attended, rising above the small copse of birch trees that almost obscured the rest of the building.

How serene everything had been years ago when the sound of the church bells would swell out in waves on Sunday morning, inundating the surrounding valley with a joyous tumult. Millie's father would swing her up on his shoulders and make a frantic effort to hold onto his hat which she invariably would strike with one of her soaring limbs. Then straddling his neck she'd squeeze his larynx and be seized with a spasm of laughter as he took her hands away saying: "Sweet child, do you want to strangle your father when he is just a mere boy in his prime?"

"You're not a boy, daddy," she'd say and her little body would again be caught in a wild spasm of giggling.

They'd start out the back door and Millie's mother would frown and call after them.

"Albert, why do you insist on going up the hill to church? You always get so muddy. You know how much it annoys me."

Her father would wave his hand at her mother, chuckling.

"You go by the road, Maud. We'll meet you there. We promise not to get muddy, don't we, dear sweet child."

They'd walk past the barns, up the grassy hill, her father's chest expanding enormously as he climbed, his hands tight on her legs.

"Why doesn't mother ever want to see us happy, daddy?"

"It's not that, dear. She just doesn't want us to get all dirty on Sunday. She wants us to be nice and clean so she can be proud of us."

But Millie knew the fierce jealousy that had developed between her and her mother. She was both frightened and puzzled by it and this caused her love for her father to become more intense.

Up the hill they'd go, along the low winding stone wall where a chipmunk now and again would nervously survey the scene and scurry away among the stones and leaves. Scattered over the field Millie saw the gray softly heaped-up disks where the cows had been.

They'd reach the church a full five minutes before her mother and wait there before the fine old stone campanile. To the far side, Millie would look at the gray monuments of the cemetery and feel a sudden tight grip on her heart. Below them on the slope opposite the farm stretched the houses of the townspeople. All the paths would be crowded with everybody walking to church. Her father would wave to the men and tip his hat to the ladies and sputter as Millie tightened her grip on his neck. All the while she sat in a haze of overwhelming joy on her father's shoulders.

Now Millie stood in the kitchen and saw that it was dark outside. Freddie had snapped on the kitchen light and she hadn't even noticed.

She turned suddenly and got her coat from the hook near the door. Freddie had finished eating and had again taken his post near the front window.

"Where are you going, Millie?" Freddie cried out. "Please don't leave me alone."

"I'll be back in a little while, Freddie," she said. "Don't worry. Everything's all right."

She was out on the soft, rich, black soil walking quietly and quickly, just like her father had done years ago. She rounded the barn and started up the hill, along the stone wall. Everything was black. She could have walked this route without faltering even if her eyes had been closed. The ground was wet and she inhaled the fullness of the soil and the grass and the heaped-up disks that the cows had dropped.

The night was punctured by the faint light of the stars. Far to her left, just above the trees, the arc of the moon thrust its upper horn into the darkness.

She reached the church and walked straight to the cemetery. There was the simple gray stone slab flush with the ground that marked her father's grave. In one quick motion she knelt and touched her lips to the cold stone. Her eyes suddenly filled with tears. Her heart beat wildly and she was breathing hard.

Again that sense of emptiness seized her and she thought, I am an empty room. She became terribly frightened. She couldn't understand why this thought kept entering her mind. There it was over and over again. It was impossible to free herself from its grip. She had a perception of disaster, a dark shadow that swamped her mind and left her trembling with fear.

She jumped up and ran from the tight enclosure of the cemetery. She saw the stone campanile of the church loom above her. She remembered the door. Opening it quickly, she entered and felt the deep stark cold of the stones. She stood there shivering in her coat in the blackness. She couldn't understand what she was doing, but she knew she had to keep moving. I am an empty room, she thought, I am an empty room. She was deathly afraid.

She looked up and felt the sudden tightness of the muscles of her neck. Up there, up very high, even though she couldn't see it clearly, she knew the bell hung above her, the huge heavy bell. For one wild moment, she saw herself pulling the bell rope in a mad frenzy, and when the clangor throbbed and swelled through the blackness and filled the night with its furious intensity, pounding in her head, the bell came hurtling down, crushing her fragile body against the stone floor.

She broke out in a cold sweat. She felt dizzy again and put out her hand to support herself against the stone wall. She turned quickly and ran out of the tower. She raced down the hill breathless. As she came around the barn she saw the soft yellow light in the kitchen. There was someone rocking in the chair and for an instant she had that tight feeling about her heart again.

"Pa," she whispered. "Pa."

She ran into the house and hugged the figure in the rocking chair. She was sobbing hysterically. She kissed him on the cheek, her eyes closed tightly, her face wet with tears.

"Pa," she whispered again.

"Millie," Freddie said. "What's the matter?"

She jumped up, suddenly aware of Freddie in the chair.

"Go to bed, Freddie," she yelled angrily.

"I'm afraid, Millie," Freddie said. He started to cry.

"There's nothing to be afraid of, Freddie. Go to bed. We've got a lot to do tomorrow."

Suddenly, Freddie was in front of her. He held her arm.

"You're sure nothing's going to happen, Millie?"

"Yes, I'm sure, Freddie. Now be good and go to bed."

Millie turned away. Freddie hugged her and kissed her on the lips. She pulled away so suddenly that Freddie jumped. Her face twisted strangely.

"Go to bed, Freddie," she said angrily, pushing him away. "I told you to go to bed. Now do as I say."

Freddie turned and walked slowly out of the room. His shoulders were held rigid and he walked stiffly, as if frightened to make any noise.

Millie stood in the middle of the kitchen, her face tight with anger. She listened to Freddie climb the stairs and then heard the floor creak above as he went slowly to his room. She felt a muscle jump in her neck. She rubbed it for a while, but it didn't stop.

She snapped off the light and sat at the kitchen table in the dark. I am an empty room, she thought. And now her eyes filled with tears that streamed down her face. Her heart seemed ready to burst out of her chest as she thought of her father again. If only he hadn't died. Then she remembered her mother. Millie's hands, wet with tears, tightened into fists in silent anger. The memory of the night her mother had run away with one of the farmhands was like a flaming image in her mind. Even then her father had said nothing. The lines in his face just deepened and his body appeared gaunt and bent with increasing fatigue. Millie was only ten years old at that time.

During the next few years, she watched helplessly as the urge to live gradually left her father.

"You have to live until I'm an old lady, Pa, because I can't handle the farm by myself, you know."

Her father would hug her.

"I figure I was built to last a hundred years, Millie. Is that long enough?"

"Maybe," Millie giggled.

Her father would kiss her.

"I don't know what I'd do without you, Millie. You're a great little housekeeper, cook, and farmhand. If I had to pay you what you're worth, I'd go broke in a week."

One night he went to sleep early, tired and exhausted as usual. He never woke up, the lines in his face finally smoothed. It was odd, she thought, how much younger her father looked in death.

Millie sat at the kitchen table in the dark for a long time. She felt stiff and tired when she finally got up and went to her room. She undressed quickly in the dark and got into bed, the springs creaking noisily. She lay there quietly, listening to Freddie turn in his bed in the next room. She knew he wasn't asleep. She could hear him breathing loudly through his mouth.

She dreaded the nights, finding it increasingly difficult to fall asleep.

She finally dozed off, turning fitfully from side to side.

Then suddenly she was wide awake again. She heard Freddie in her room and she sat up quickly, the covers falling from her heaving chest.

"Freddie, what are you doing here? What's the matter?"

Freddie knelt by her bed. He was crying and terrible sobs shuddered through his body.

"Freddie, what's the matter?" Millie said again softly.

She reached out and her hand touched his hot wet face. She drew back quickly.

"Freddie," she said.

"Millie, what're we going to do?"

His crying was terrible, his whole body shaking. She wanted to cover her ears, to block out the bells that started banging in her head, to block out his voice that sounded so much like her father.

"Go to bed, Freddie," she said. "I told you that everything is going to be all right."

Her voice shook. Her whole body trembled.

"Is it, Millie, honest?" Freddie said. "Is it really?"

"Yes, Freddie," she said. "Now go to bed."

"I can't sleep, Millie."

He reached out and touched her side with his wet fingers. Her flesh suddenly leaped beneath his hand.

"Freddie," she said again softly.

"I don't think I'll ever sleep again, Millie," Freddie said.

He was no longer crying. His voice took on a strange intensity. His hands moved again in the dark and she felt their hot wetness on her breasts.

"No, Freddie," she said.

Her whole body leaped beneath his hands. She shuddered in a prolonged spasm and then was stiff like wood.

I am an empty room, she thought. She felt Freddie holding her tightly. She started to cry silently. Her chest hurt and she kept feeling Freddie's hands wet with tears on her body.

Her whole flesh kept leaping wildly and yet oddly, she felt stiff as wood.

"Millie, Millie, you're crying," Freddie said.

She felt his fingers tighten on her until she wanted to cry out in pain.

After a while she felt cold and dead. Freddie had fallen asleep by her side and she lay there listening to his deep regular breathing. She couldn't move. A shudder gripped her body now and again as she lay still, hardly daring to breathe.

She knew what she had to do. There was nobody to take care of Freddie when she was gone. She didn't want to leave the warmth of the bed. She could hear the bells banging in her head again.

She finally got up and left the room.

The last thing Freddie remembered was Millie almost like dead at his side. He was frightened but was too tired to do anything except lie there.

He didn't know how long he had slept . He woke up suddenly and called out Millie's name. It was still dark and he couldn't see anything in the room.

"Millie," he called out again.

He kept looking around. He finally made out a dark figure in the doorway.

"Is that you, Millie? What're you doing?"

"It's me, Freddie. Don't worry. Everything is going to be all right. I promised you, didn't I?"

"Yes, Millie, you did," Freddie said.

There was a loud blast as Millie squeezed the trigger of her father's shotgun. A long flame leaped out towards Freddie. He didn't make a sound.

Millie threw the gun to the floor. She heard the bells banging in her head, heavy metallic tones that swelled and throbbed within her skull. The whole room reverberated with the crashing and she felt the whole earth tremble and move about.

She turned slowly and walked down the stairs, out of the house and past the barns. She felt the coldness of the black wet soil against her bare feet and smelled the sweet smell of hay. All about her as she walked, she heard the wild tumult of the bells in the night, banging inside her skull, almost jubilant in their madness. She felt the cold damp air against her skin but it didn't bother her.

"Pa," she said, "I know you'll understand."

She breathed hard as she walked up the hill along the winding stone wall up through the copse of birch trees to the campanile of the church.

The faint light of the moon cast a weird pattern of shadows

across the small clearing. She walked to her father's grave. She bent down and kissed the stone.

"Pa," she said again, "I had to do it. There was no other way."

She walked back to the bell tower. The sound of the bells was like a giant hammer smashing against her brain. Her whole body seemed to vibrate to their swelling tones. She walked inside and stood there without moving. She finally stepped forward groping for the rope. She looked up. The bells were faintly visible. They were not moving but she still heard their wild clangor in her skull. She found a chair in the dark and placed it beneath the rope. She began to pull on the rope, making the bells ring out, slowly at first, then louder in a violent riotous agitation. The sounds in her head stopped as soon as the bells in the tower rang out.

She climbed up on the chair, tied the end of the rope around her neck, and jumped.

LESSONS TO BE LEARNED

Millie had developed an abnormal attachment to her father; and when he died, her grieving progressed to a deep depression. Insomnia and severe headaches are prominent symptoms of depression, two clues missed by her physician. She sought help from a doctor who was too busy to listen, one who preferred to deal in superficialities, and Millie was too depressed to realize she was seeking help from the wrong physician. She instead came to the conclusion there was nobody who could help her. Her depression had imprisoned her in an inescapable web of hopelessness. When she was finally cornered by the forced sale of her father's farm and cows, she rejected Mr. Kendall's silent offer and solved her problem in her own tragic way.

Physicians complain that neither insurance companies nor Medicare pays a physician to listen. This is not a valid excuse to turn away from a patient who needs help. All physicians have been taught to listen long enough to enable them to arrive at a proper diagnosis. The history taken by a physician is frequently more important than the actual physical examination, especially early in a disease process.

In psychiatric cases, the depth of depression can be difficult to assess. And unfortunately, many physicians avoid asking patients directly whether they have ever contemplated suicide.

There is no doubt that Millie could have been helped by a more astute and attentive physician. The clues were there for both the doctor and the patient. The doctor was too busy and the patient too depressed, so Millie left the physician's office convinced there was no way out of her dilemma except by taking the tragic path to self-destruction.

Chapter Eight

An Emergency

Stanley Truhart started his rendezvous with death at 6:00 a.m. He awoke with severe upper abdominal pain radiating into his chest. He turned a ghastly white and immediately broke out with a cold sweat as his blood pressure dropped precipitously. His wife called 911 and he was taken to the emergency room of a community hospital where I was on staff.

The doctor on duty, sensing a catastrophic event, then made his first mistake. Instead of performing a brief but thorough exam, he felt the patient's belly and quickly called one of the senior attending surgeons, who happened to be in the E.R. seeing another patient for a minor problem. The surgeon examined Truhart's belly, noted the blood pressure taken by the nurse to be 70/40 with a pulse of 120, and made the diagnosis of a ruptured aortic aneurysm (a tear in a weakened ballooned-out area of the major blood vessel coursing down the back of the abdomen).

An EKG was done quickly and left unread on the counter. Blood was drawn and the patient was then rushed to the operating room.

I had just finished my rounds and was about to drive to my office for morning hours when I heard my name called out by the page operator. The E.R. was calling to advise me that my patient was on his way to the operating room with a ruptured aneurysm and that there was no time for me to see the patient even though I had been in the hospital for the last two hours.

About thirty minutes later, the patient's wife called and asked me if I had seen her husband in the E.R. I told her I hadn't, and that I had been merely notified that her husband had been taken to the operating room for immediate surgery.

She asked me to look in on her husband after the surgery had been completed, which I agreed to do.

About eleven o'clock, I drove back to the hospital and happened to see the surgeon just as he was about to leave.

"How is Stanley Truhart?" I said.

"Oh, is he your patient? He's holding his own, that's about all I can say at the moment. He's in the recovery room if you want to see him."

Stanley Truhart was not holding his own. He appeared to be dying. I looked through the notes in his chart. The surgeon having found no blood in his abdomen, and no evidence of a ruptured aneurysm, then explored the abdominal cavity thoroughly. On palpation of the gall bladder, he noted multiple gall stones. He proceeded to excise the gall bladder, feeling that it would be a shame to do nothing in the presence of a gall bladder full of stones.

"Do you have Mr. Truhart's EKG?" I asked the nurse at the desk.

"No," she said. "It was done in the E.R. but probably is in the EKG room now waiting to be read by a cardiologist."

It was scheduled to be returned to the patient's chart the next day. Just in time for the autopsy, I supposed.

The lab work gave no clue to the patient's moribund condition. I walked quickly to the EKG lab. The young technician there had some difficulty finding the tracing. This was not unusual in our hospital. If it hadn't been an emergency, the EKG would have been found immediately. The more you need something in a hurry, the longer it takes to find—Murphy's Law.

"It hasn't been officially read yet," she said, after locating it under a large pile of unread tracings.

There was the answer on the tracing in my hand. It revealed an acute anterior myocardial infarction, a severe heart attack involving the major blood vessel on the front side of the heart.

"When was this taken?" I asked the nurse.

"The time is on the tracing, I believe, Doctor. Yes, here it is, in the E.R. at 6:20 a.m., just before he was rushed to surgery."

So here was poor Stanley Truhart, experiencing an overwhelming heart attack involving the left anterior descending coronary artery, the main vessel supplying blood to the heart, misdiagnosed in the emergency room as a ruptured aorta by an overly-eager surgeon and then subjected to a major surgical procedure, an exploratory, followed by an unnecessary cholecystectomy. By the time he got to his room in the Intensive Care Unit, he appeared to have suffered the worst kind of mob-mugging a person could have experienced in New York's Central Park. And worst of all, he was obligated to pay for all this unnecessary treatment to the tune of twenty-five thousand dollars and his life.

I called the cardiologist immediately. Even with heroic measures, the patient continued on his relentless course with his rendezvous with death. He expired approximately twelve hours after surgery.

"We did everything we could for your husband, Mrs. Truhart," the surgeon said that evening to the widow.

"Thank you, Doctor," Mrs. Truhart said, crying.

She turned to leave, tears flowing down both cheeks, but then stopped and turned back to the surgeon, who looked uncomfortable and eager to depart.

"Do you think an autopsy would provide any useful information to me and my children, Doctor?" she said, half sobbing.

"No, I don't think so," the surgeon said. "Your husband has suffered enough. We should let him rest in peace."

"You've been so kind to us throughout this ordeal, Doctor," Mrs. Truhart said. "I don't know how to thank you. God bless you."

LESSONS TO BE LEARNED

It is difficult to think of a greater mistake than the one in this chapter. A great and dazzling ego is involved, one that refused consultation of any kind.

There is no doubt that speed is important once the diagnosis of a leaking or ruptured aneurysm is established. Every second counts. But haste isn't so important that it excuses an improper diagnosis. A nurse could have rushed the EKG to any cardiologist or internist in the hospital and a quick reading could have prevented this debacle.

Once the surgeon was inside the abdomen and suddenly realized he had made the wrong diagnosis, he should have gotten out immediately, especially when he knew the patient was in shock prior to surgery. An acute gall bladder attack doesn't cause the patient to go into shock and break out in a cold sweat.

The surgeon overlooked the most common cause of this clinical picture: an acute, myocardial infarction. Instead, on exploring the abdomen, he found a gall bladder full of stones and thoughtlessly proceeded to excise it, thereby prolonging the anesthesia by two hours. A good history would have revealed the patient had never suffered a gall bladder attack in spite of his gall stones. A "silent" gall bladder such as this doesn't require surgery.

The patient's wife, by not demanding an autopsy, let the surgeon off the hook. It's true that a malpractice suit will not bring a patient back to life, but she had an obligation to her husband to determine the specific diagnosis. Initially, she had been told her husband had suffered a ruptured aortic aneurysm. Why, then, was his gall bladder taken out? Was she even told about this procedure? There's no doubt that grief can render a family mute, but certain questions must be asked ultimately.

PATIENT BEWARE—

Later on, when she had read the death certificate, she called me to ask when her husband had suffered the heart attack. She thought the surgery might have caused it. I told her it had occurred at home when her husband first woke up with chest pain. I thought the cardiologist had previously discussed this with her. Perhaps he had and in the turmoil she had forgotten about it. She thanked me and I never heard from her again.

The surgeon was never reprimanded.

Chapter Nine

The Lump

Ray Larkin was a tall, handsome, blue-eyed, black-haired Irishman. He was born with the customary Irish charm, but a charm so natural and so infused with sincerity that everybody liked him the moment they met him. He had a big booming voice and a laugh to match. When Ray laughed, all of us in our small, medical school class were inclined to laugh with him.

He wasn't laughing, however, when Dr. Cornelius Stiles grasped his scrotum in his right hand, during our annual physical examination in our first year of medical school, and said quietly, "You have a lump in your epididymis, Dr. Larkin."

"In my what?" Ray said.

"Your epididymis," Dr. Stiles said. "That's a cord-like structure, a tube, on the posterior aspect of the testis where sperm are stored. It's coiled just like a telephone cord. There is a small lump just as the epididymis comes out of the testis."

"Is it something serious?" Ray said, looking worried.

"It could be. But it also could be something as simple as a previous infection that left a scar in your epididymis."

"What kind of an infection?" Ray said.

"Gonorrhea," Dr. Stiles said. "Do you have a history of gonorrhea?"

"No," Ray said, "but while I was in the service I had some aching in my scrotum and I think the final diagnosis was acute epididymitis. I was treated with a sulfa drug. I had forgotten all about it."

"That's the most likely cause of your problem, a urinary tract infection. It left a little scarred-up lump in your epididymis at the base of your testis."

"What do I have to do?" Ray said.

"We'll check it out when you have your annual physical exam next year at the school. I wouldn't worry about it. It's merely a historical landmark of your past activities."

Ray laughed his dirty laugh but it wasn't convincing. He told everybody in the class about his problem and that seemed to relieve any anxiety he may have had. If Dr. Stiles wasn't worried about it, there was no sense for him to worry about it either.

We were exceptionally busy in the first year of medical school so Ray's lump was soon forgotten.

But at the beginning of our second year, we had another physical examination, and the lump was still there on palpation of the scrotum.

"Your lump is unchanged, I'm glad to say, Dr. Larkin," Dr. Stiles said. "If it had been a cancer it certainly would have gotten larger by now."

"You're not worried that it could be a cancer, are you, Dr. Stiles?"

"The fact that it hasn't grown at all in the past year indicates its benign nature. You have nothing to worry about except your exams in medical school. You can forget about this lump."

Ray was happy and he broadcast the good news to the entire class.

In the spring of our second year, we were studying various pathological conditions, including skin lesions. Ray began to worry about some of the dark brown spots he had on his back. One day in histology, he pulled up his shirt in class and turned to the man sitting next to him.

"What do you think of this one, Tom, the one my finger is on?"

Tom Slater looked at it very carefully. He had Ray turn back and forth in front of the window.

"Hm-m-m," Tom said.

"Well, come on, come on," Ray said, "we haven't got all day."

"Well," Tom said, dragging the word out to a full sentence. "In my considered opinion, and based on my vast knowledge in this field, you have only twenty-four hours to live. So hand over the keys to your car. I have a hot date this weekend."

Ray was taking no chances. A few days later, he had three benign melanomas excised from his back. He told the surgeon he was worried they might be malignant. The surgeon reassured him of their benign nature, but Ray insisted that they be excised.

"You can have the sutures removed when you return here after spring vacation or you can have your own doctor remove them in one week while you're home," the surgeon said.

Before Ray came back to school, he made an appointment with a surgeon in New York who was a friend of his family. While he was there having his skin sutures removed, Ray happened to mention the lump in his epididymis. The surgeon decided to check that too.

"Ray, that is a cancer growing in your testes and it must be removed immediately."

"But Dr. Stiles said the lump was from an old urinary tract infection I had in the service," Ray said.

"Dr. Stiles is wrong," the surgeon said. "Not only do you have to have that testes removed but you also have to have a periaortic lymph node dissection to see if the cancer has spread up to your kidneys. That's the bad news. Luckily, we also have some good news. This type of cancer is most likely a seminoma and is very responsive to radiation so I can guarantee that it won't kill you."

Ray decided to have the entire procedure done at the medical school. He joked about losing one of his most valuable possessions, but we all knew he was scared to death. The entire class was waiting for him to come out of the recovery room. He was crying as the orderly wheeled the stretcher to his room.

"They cut me like an old fish," he said. "Just like an old fish. I'll never be the same."

The cancer had spread to the lymph nodes all the way up to his kidneys.

When he recovered enough from his surgery, he was sent to Boston for radiotherapy. He was told that he would never be able to have children. He subsequently made a complete recovery.

He graduated from medical school with all the rest of us and became a very successful endocrinologist in New York. Over the next ten years, he fathered two sets of twins, and an extra boy and girl for good measure, just to prove that when a physician makes a statement about the future, he is often wrong.

We saw each other every five years at our school reunions. As he grew older, his voice deepened, and his laugh sounded dirtier than ever. He became a chain smoker. He wouldn't have been recognized without a cigarette dangling from his mouth. He still had that old Irish charm and everybody liked him more than ever. Just by himself he made our class reunions happy and joyful occurrences.

At the age of forty-two, while fishing in his boat, he suddenly collapsed with a heart attack. He was taken off the boat in a coast guard helicopter and was in the hospital within twenty minutes.

He was the first one to die in our medical school class. We all felt we had lost a brother.

LESSONS TO BE LEARNED

Again we see the delayed diagnosis, the trap of being involved in "watchful waiting and careful observation." Is this really good medical care? Furthermore, the original premise was wrong. Medicine is full of red herrings and the history of a previous urinary tract infection led to a wrong conclusion. That type of thinking traps you. All physicians are trained in the task of developing a differential diagnosis. When you arrive at a diagnosis you must ask yourself a simple question: what else could it be? Too many physicians forget those five words.

It's true that sometimes physicians intervene too quickly. In this case surgical intervention was delayed far too long. The lesson here is that if you as a patient are going to be involved in "careful, watchful observation" over a period of time, you must insist on a second opinion. And if both physicians concur, you must be sure that it truly is "careful, watchful observation" and not just a lengthy period of neglect.

As for physicians making prophecies, as in this case predicting that Ray Larkin would be sterile and childless, in my experience these medical prophets are wrong more often than right.

Fortunately, seminomas are slow growing compared to other tumors. They are the most common of all testicular cancers. There is an increased incidence in patients with undescended testes. If untreated, seminomas spread upward to the iliac and periaortic lymph nodes before generalized metastases are detectable. Fortunately too, seminomas are usually extremely sensitive to radiotherapy, while other testicular tumors are not.

Survival rates are high, frequently up to 95%, if proper treatment is provided at an early stage of the disease.

PATIENT BEWARE—

But who can state that massive radiation doesn't increase the aging process, rendering the patient susceptible to a host of other degenerative problems and malignancies? Add the effects of heavy smoking (two packs or more per day) that causes a rapid increase in the development of arteriosclerosis (first demonstrated in rabbits around 1900) and we end up with a 42-year-old male with an 82-year-old heart.

Chapter Ten

A Simple Error

My brother-in-law, Jim Jameson, called me from New Brunswick.

"I'm dying," he said, "and I hope you can help me."

It was 1957. Jim was thirty-seven years old. He was a pharmacist in St. John, New Brunswick. He had been in good health until he came down with a severe, unrelenting headache that felt as if an explosion had occurred inside his head. He went to his physician immediately, fearing an impending stroke. His blood pressure was extremely high, 280/140, and was unresponsive to the common medications used at that time. Within a short time after the onset of his malignant hypertension, his vision began to fail. The headaches persisted with maximum intensity, and he was in imminent danger of suffering a massive stroke. He was admitted to a hospital in his locality for immediate surgery.

"Since we haven't been able to lower your blood pressure medically," his physician said, "we are left with only one option, a bilateral thoracolumbar sympathectomy."

He went on to explain that this involved severing a chain of nerves that control the caliber and muscle tone of blood vessels. The theory was that these arteries were in spasm from an excessive discharge from the sympathetic nervous system, resulting in severe hypertension. Once these nerves were cut, the arteries would dilate and the blood pressure would drop.

PATIENT BEWARE—

The surgery was done and Jim did improve. His blood pressure dropped but not to completely normal levels. The headaches lessened in intensity and he was able to return to work. The surgeon had told him that the benefit would only be temporary, and would last about two years. It was exactly two years after the surgery that the headaches returned with full intensity and his blood pressure rose to its previous level.

There was no response to oral medication and his future appeared grim.

I arranged to have him admitted to a hospital in Boston.

"They are doing a great deal of experimental work on this problem in Boston, and I'm sure they'll be able to control your blood pressure, Jim," I said.

I tried to appear optimistic but I knew that I wasn't fooling Jim in any way regarding the gravity of his condition.

My wife and I picked him up at the airport and drove him to the hospital. We met Dr. Lorenzo Brown, the Chief of Medicine, who was going to be Jim's physician. Dr. Brown was strictly an academic type of physician. He was cold and unemotional. It was clear to all of us that he was not going to think of Jim as anything but another number on a hospital chart. I was already regretting Jim's admission. I could almost hear Dr. Brown saying to the chief resident, "Place him on Protocol #3." And that would probably be the end of his involvement with the case.

"Malignant hypertension is a difficult disease to treat," Dr. Brown said in a flat monotone as if he were lecturing a third-year class of medical students. "Most of the patients with this problem complain of blurred vision, severe headaches, and shortness of breath. The blood pressure is usually far above 110 diastolic and frequently up to 140 to 180. Usually we find an enlarged heart and even early signs of heart failure. The eye findings are conspicuous with swelling of the optic nerve and scattered cotton wool spots. About half the patients have chronic kidney disease with raised blood urea and serum creatinine levels. There is necrosis of renal arterioles because of the inability of the kidneys to adjust to the high blood pressure. A similar change occurs in the retina with flame-like hemorrhages that can be easily visualized with the ophthalmoscope. The same process occurs in the brain with swelling of the brain tissue and leakage of plasma into the surrounding areas."

He certainly didn't have to go to this extent to impress us with his knowledge of the disease process that was killing my brother-in-law. We assumed Dr. Brown knew what he had to know about malignant hypertension and the proper treatment.

"Do you mind if I sit down, Dr. Brown?" Jim said, interrupting the flat monotone.

"Not at all, Mr. Jameson," Dr. Brown said. "Now in your case, we plan to start you on a new and powerful ganglionic blocker, called Inversine. I'll be checking you every day myself because of the nature of the drug. It requires extreme care in its titration."

He turned to me.

"Are you familiar with this medication, Doctor?"

"Yes," I said, "as a matter of fact, I am. I have three patients with severe hypertension who were unresponsive to other milder drugs. After attending a symposium on Inversine, I started them on this medication and they have done remarkably well."

"No family physician should be using Inversine, Doctor," he said. "You'll have to excuse me but I have to tell you it is much too powerful to be used outside of the hospital by nonspecialists. It must be started in the hospital under very strict conditions controlled by specialists in the field of hypertension."

"That is exactly how I use it," I said. "I start the patients in the hospital, being careful to check the BUN and the creatinine, so as not to precipitate kidney failure. Once they are stabilized, with blood pressures taken in the standing position, I then discharge them and restabilize them on an outpatient basis."

"I'm afraid you're going to get into a whole lot of trouble using that drug, Doctor. Sooner or later, some patient is going to accuse you of precipitating renal failure, even though this may be the end result of this disease. I hope you don't mind me giving you a little piece of friendly advice as one physician to another."

"On the contrary, Dr. Brown. I appreciate your comments."

Dr. Brown told Jim to write down any questions that he might have regarding the treatment protocol. He promised to answer them during the week. We handed Jim's records to Dr. Brown and then remained with Jim until he was settled in his room.

"I'll call you every day, Jim," I said. "If you need anything, please let us know."

The next day, Jim gave me a brief summary of his day.

"The nurses are wonderful," he said, "but the doctors are too busy."

"What do you mean?" I said.

"They poke one foot in the door while reading the chart, ask me how I'm doing, and leave before I can even answer them."

"Do the doctors take your blood pressure?" I said.

"No, only the nurses," he said.

"Well, the next time a doctor sticks his head in the door, make sure you ask him to take your blood pressure."

When I called the next day, I asked Jim if he had been successful in getting a doctor to take his blood pressure."

"One of the students took it," he said. "Every time I stand up, I faint. So the nurse has been nice to me and takes my blood pressure while I lie flat on my back."

"Are you getting your Inversine around the clock?" I said.

"Oh sure," he said. "I'm getting the full dose."

"Jim, listen to me," I said. "While you're on Inversine, they have to take your blood pressure with you standing up. If you faint, or your blood pressure drops precipitously, the next dose is either skipped or reduced, depending on the drop in blood pressure. Ask them for an Inversine package insert so that you can become familiar with this medication. It can cause renal failure, you know. Has Dr. Brown been in to see you since your admission?"

"Not yet," he said.

I tried to phone Dr. Brown several times but he never returned the calls. Jim was discharged one week later and told to remain on his Inversine medication, An intern was the only one to see him on the day of his discharge. Dr. Brown did not see him during his entire hospitalization.

We picked him up and drove him back to Connecticut. We were not at all happy with his Boston hospitalization. The first thing I did when we got back home was check his blood pressure. Standing up it was zero. That was the reason he fainted. Lying down it was just as high as it had been before admission. That was the reason he had been getting the full dose of Inversine. I drew his blood to check his BUN. This is the level of nitrogenous waste products in the blood and is a good indicator of kidney function. I already knew it was going to be higher.

On admission, his BUN was 48 mgm%. The normal level is 9 to 18. This is the number of milligrams per 100 cubic centimeters of blood. On the day I took him home, his BUN was 148 mgm%, indicating a dramatic drop in renal function. I suspected what was obvious, that kidney failure had been precipitated by improper use of Inversine.

I immediately stopped the drug and put him on a low protein diet to take the pressure off his kidneys. His BUN began to drop slowly over the next few days and he began to feel slightly better. But he knew he was dying, and he was eager to get back home. Dialysis was not clinically available at that time. Jim knew there was nothing more to be done for him.

We drove back to the airport and put him on the plane to New Brunswick, knowing in our hearts that this was probably the last time we would see him alive.

A few days later, Dr. Brown called me from Boston.

"Is your brother-in-law still alive?"

"Yes, he is," I said, "but he doesn't look like he's going to last more than a few weeks."

I told him about the change in the BUN.

"I have a confession to make to you," he said.

"Yes?" I said. I already knew what he was going to say.

"I thought the chief medical resident was checking the blood pressure on your brother-in-law. He thought the intern was doing it. The truth of the matter is that the nurse was the only one taking his blood pressure. Every time he stood up, his blood pressure dropped to zero, and he would faint. The nurse took pity on him and allowed him to lie flat in bed when she recorded his pressure, with the result that the readings were all too high. He got the full dose of Inversine each time and that caused his renal failure."

There was a long silence on the phone after his confession.

"Didn't you give me a lecture on that very subject, Dr. Brown, on the day my brother-in-law was admitted?" I said.

"Yes, I remember doing that," he said. "I feel like a complete ass, sad but wiser."

I hung up the phone without saying another word.

Back in New Brunswick, Jim was too sick to go to work. His physician had put him back on Inversine and his BUN continued to rise. He was dying from uremia. He developed inflammation of the membrane around his heart, a condition called pericarditis, and he was suffering severe chest pains. He was still at home when my wife called him a few days later. He was too weak to come to the phone. I called his physician and he was immediately hospitalized.

The headaches were much worse, and the pain from his pericarditis that had started out intermittently and stabbing in nature, became continuous. His brother, Teddy, was there trying to comfort him. He called the nurse to give Jim something for the pain.

"I'm sorry," the nurse said. "Mr. Jameson's doctor did not leave any orders for pain medication."

"Well, call the intern or the resident," Teddy said.

"We don't have any interns or residents," the nurse said.

"Then call my brother's doctor immediately. He has to have something for pain. It's unbearable."

The nurse came back a few minutes later.

"The doctor is not answering his page," she said, looking genuinely upset.

Teddy sat down on the bed and held Jim in his arms. Jim took a deep breath and died.

LESSONS TO BE LEARNED

Malignant hypertension is an example of accelerated hypertension. Today with widespread early treatment of this problem with a variety of efficacious drugs, it is no longer seen as frequently as it was 30-40 years ago. It is most commonly seen after the age of 40, but Jim Jameson was only 35 years old when he developed this devastating disease and he was dead in 2 years.

Malignant hypertension is basically high pressure autoregulatory failure with severe damage in target organs such as the kidneys, heart, and brain. If the blood pressure rises slowly over a period of years, as it does frequently in the elderly, autoregulatory failure doesn't occur as the body gradually adapts to the slowly rising pressure. Because of this, malignant hypertension is rarely seen in the elderly.

The problem illustrated in this chapter happens too often in large university medical centers. The superspecialist, so involved with events of a loftier nature and so habituated to speaking from the top of the mountain to the lowly, ignorant masses, just happens to forget his obligations to the miserable soul who comes to seek his good and kindly ministrations.

Once I sent a patient to a big university medical center consultant who didn't even bother to see the patient at all. He turned him over to a resident who then passed himself off as a member of the consulting staff.

In this particular case, with a fulminating malignant hypertension, it was undoubtedly true that nothing much could have been done for the patient at that specific point in time. But that is no excuse for robbing the patient of even one day of his life. A doctor must remember at all times: *physician, do no harm*. Today, with the arsenal of powerful and often deadly medications and treatments at the physician's disposal, it's important to remember that restriction more than ever. It's especially unforgivable after the "super-physician" allows his ego to render a dissertation to a lowly family physician on proper care of the patient and then neglects to follow his own instructions.

Chapter Eleven

The Doubter

"You better come up and see my wife, Doc," Tom Marsh cackled over the phone in his high-pitched voice. "She's terribly sick."

"What's the problem, Tom?"

"I don't know. She was all right until a few minutes ago. She started to wash the dishes and all of a sudden she got dizzy and turned white. You'd better hurry. She looks like she's going to die."

Tom rarely got this excited so I knew that I'd better get there quickly, even though I thought it may very well turn out to be nothing more than a fainting spell.

When I got to his house, his wife Della was lying on the couch appearing totally exsanguinated. She was completely white, as if every drop of blood had been removed from her body.

"What happened, Della?" I said as I knelt beside the couch to take her blood pressure.

"I was washing dishes, Doctor. I couldn't eat much of anything because my stomach has been bothering me. All of a sudden, I got dizzy and nearly fell over. Tom helped me to the couch and called you right away."

Her voice was very weak. Her blood pressure was 74/52, and her pulse was racing at 140. Her chest was clear. Her heart was beating rapidly but otherwise did not sound unusual.

"When did your stomach start to bother you, Della?"

"Only since I fell and hurt my back two weeks ago. Do you think it could be the pain medicine Dr. Keller gave me for my back strain?"

On examination, her belly was rigid. Every quadrant of her abdomen was board-like to palpation, due to massive muscle spasm, a sign of a surgical belly. There seemed to be a greater amount of spasm in the left upper quadrant in the vicinity of her spleen.

"I don't think so, Della. Did you injure your belly when you fell?"

"I just slipped on some ice when I tried to open the garage door. Only my back hurt. I went to see Dr. Keller in Morrisville. You know him, he's a surgeon. He told me I strained my back. With heat and rest, he said I'd be better in a few days. What do you think is wrong, Doctor?"

"Apparently, you tore your spleen in that fall two weeks ago, Della, and it's been bleeding off and on since then. I'll call Dr. Keller and see if he can meet us at the emergency room of the hospital. I'm not going to wait for the ambulance. I'll take you up myself."

Luckily, Dr. Keller answered his page immediately.

"What's up, Ed," he said.

"I've got your patient, Della Marsh, here at her home and I believe she has a torn spleen. She's in shock and I'm going to take her to the hospital myself. Will you wait there for us? I believe she'll need immediate surgery and blood."

"OK," Dr. Keller said, "but I doubt that she has a ruptured spleen. You know, I saw her just two weeks ago right after she fell. She hasn't reinjured herself, has she?"

"No," I said, "but I think she has been bleeding off and on since her fall."

"I doubt that," Dr. Keller said, "but bring her up and I'll take a look at her."

Dr. Keller was there in the emergency room waiting for us. He examined Della while the lab technician drew her blood.

"Well, what do you think?" I said.

"I'll tell you after I do a few more studies. First, we'll get some blood started."

"Call me after you do the surgery, Jack, and let me know what you find. I'll be at the office." I looked at my watch. "I'm late already."

It was an exceptionally busy afternoon and I didn't get any free time until 4:30. I still hadn't heard from Dr. Keller so I had him paged at the hospital.

"Well, what did you find at surgery, Jack?" I said.

"I haven't gone in yet," he said.

"What!"

I couldn't believe that he hadn't even started.

"What's taking so long?" I said.

"As soon as Dr. Quinn finishes closing her up, I'll go in and take out her spleen."

"What the hell is Dr. Quinn doing in there? He's a gynecologist!"

"My diagnosis was a ruptured ovary and I called him in to do a laparotomy. Her ovaries are normal. It's a ruptured spleen. We've been pumping blood into her all afternoon."

I could hardly restrain myself. I felt like telling him that he was lucky that the patient was still alive.

About one hour later, Dr. Keller finally went in and took out her spleen. There was a small tear in it that just kept pumping out blood. Spleens are notorious for bleeding off and on for days after a seemingly minor injury until they reach a point where so much blood has been lost that immediate surgery is necessary to save the patient.

Della Marsh was a strong lady and had been in good health until this accident. For three days she improved rapidly. She then developed a deep thrombophlebitis of her lower extremities. A few days after that, she suffered a pulmonary embolus in spite of being on anticoagulants. A clot had torn loose from the veins in her legs and had lodged in her lungs. She gradually recovered from those two setbacks and just as she was about ready for discharge, she developed a fulminating pneumonia.

She spent a total of six weeks in the hospital recovering from her post-operative complications. I saw her briefly on the day she was discharged.

"Isn't Dr. Keller wonderful?" she said smiling. "He saved my life."

"Yes, he is," I said.

I mentioned her case to Joe Davis, Dr. Keller's partner.

"Jack Keller is a stubborn mule," he said. "If you send him a case with a tentative diagnosis, he'll do his damndest to prove you're wrong. What he did with that ruptured spleen was inexcusable. It's amazing that she survived."

About one month later, I had another interesting case that led to another encounter with Dr. Keller. Tony Markley walked into the office without an appointment. I had seen him before for a few minor, insignificant problems, but he was not a man who came to the office eagerly.

"You got to do something with my stomach, Doc. It's been aching like all hell."

"How long has it been hurting, Tony?" I said.

"It doesn't hurt, Doc. It just aches. It's been aching for a week. I've been painting ceilings and I must have strained my belly muscles. Can you give me something for strained muscles?"

"Well, get up on the examining table and let's see what a good diagnostician you are."

He had a rigid abdomen, totally board-like. By careful palpation, it seemed that the problem was localized in the right lower quadrant, where the appendix is located. This was where the maximum spasm appeared to be. He also had rebound pain in that area. By palpating the opposite side and then releasing the pressure, the patient experiences pain over the inflamed area. These are the typical findings in acute appendicitis. However, in a ruptured appendix, the abdomen becomes board-like, making palpation more difficult to evaluate. Intestinal peristalsis stops, so on auscultation of the abdomen (listening with the stethoscope), there are no bowel sounds.

"Tony," I said, "it appears that you have a ruptured appendix. I'm going to send you to the hospital immediately."

"Now hold on, Doc," Tony Markley said. "It's not a ruptured appendix and I'm not going to any hospital to have some dang fool surgeon open me up just because he needs a little more money to go on vacation. All I need is some medicine for these strained muscles. How could a man walk around for a week with a ruptured appendix?"

"He could if he was a stubborn mule like you are, Tony. All right, let's compromise. Go to the lab and get a CBC, a complete blood count."

"What's that going to show us?" he said.

"The normal white blood cell count is about 4500 to 11000. In the presence of infection like a ruptured appendix, the count rises dramatically, up to 18000 and higher. I'll bet that yours is going to be over 18000. If it is, you're going to the hospital whether you like it or not. Of course, I could always call your daughter if you get too stubborn for me to handle."

"Jesus," he said. "Don't do that. I'll go to the lab."

Tony was back in twenty minutes. His white count was 24000.

"Now, what surgeon would you like me to call?"

"I just don't understand it, Doc, honest. Walking around with a ruptured appendix for a whole week. Call Dr. Keller, if you really think you have to, but I just don't understand it at all."

Jack Keller, of all people, I thought. What did I do to deserve this?

I caught him just as he was about to leave the hospital.

"I'm sending a patient by the name of Tony Markley up to the emergency room right away. He's been walking around with a ruptured appendix for a week. He thought his belly was sore from painting ceilings."

"Send him right up. I'll wait for him, but I have to tell you, I doubt very much that he has a ruptured appendix if he's been walking around painting ceilings all week."

No, not again, I thought.

"Well, this patient doesn't have ovaries, so you won't have to call Dr. Quinn this time," I said.

"Smart-ass," he said, and slammed down the receiver.

Dr. Keller didn't bother to call me back with his findings at surgery and I decided it was senseless to call him.

Three months later, Tony Markley came into the office with a sore throat. He didn't have an appointment this time, either. I examined him and the nurse did a throat smear for beta hemolytic strep, which was positive. I gave him a prescription for penicillin and told him to take it for ten days even though he would start feeling much better in two or three.

"Now, aren't you going to tell me what happened three months ago when I sent you to the emergency room to see Dr. Keller?" I said.

"Oh sure," he said. "Didn't Dr. Keller call you?"

"No, he didn't," I said.

"Well, you were right, it was a ruptured appendix. Dr. Keller said anybody could have made that diagnosis with a blood count that high."

"Keep talking," I said.

"He examined me and then repeated the blood count, because he didn't trust outside labs, he said. Then he told me to go home and to take nothing by mouth except water and not even that after midnight. He gave me instructions to be at the hospital at eight o'clock in the morning and I was there on the dot. He operated on me but couldn't take out the appendix. There was too much pus, so he just drained it. He told me that in a few months, he would put me back in the hospital and take out the appendix, after all the inflammation is gone. I tell you, Doctor, he's got a long wait if he's waiting for me."

I'll go along with that, I muttered under my breath as Tony left the room.

I never sent another patient to Dr. Keller.

LESSONS TO BE LEARNED

This surgeon happened to be a good technician but for some unknown reason had to go to great lengths to disprove the diagnoses of his referring physicians. By his stubbornness, he delayed proper medical care. I suppose with lumps and bumps and hernias, he was probably trustworthy. But serious cases should never be sent to this type of individual. This certainly doesn't mean he has to accept the opinions of referring physicians as gospel. It just means that he has to keep an open mind. This is a simple requirement but very difficult to observe by individuals who are so impressed with themselves that they allow their egos to penetrate the ozone layer.

How can a patient recognize a surgeon with an ego impediment of such monstrous proportions? It's not easy but it can be done. The first clue is when the surgeon criticizes the diagnosis of the referring physician and then finds it to be correct. The second clue is the stormy post-operative course of the patient. There is no doubt that poor surgery leads to all sorts of deadly complications. You must understand, however, that even good surgery can have its share of poor results. Many of the best surgeons operate on more high-risk patients and that factor alone leads to rough post-operative courses.

In the first case, we can ask if the delayed surgery directly caused the many complications this patient suffered. That question would be difficult to answer. But we can definitely say that subjecting her to a useless operative procedure requiring 2-3 hours of anesthesia certainly did not help her.

Della Marsh remained loyal to her surgeon in spite of her stormy post-operative course. She even survived the shock of receiving a surgical bill from the gynecologist. She believed Dr. Keller had saved her life and I wouldn't have tried to change her mind. However, I wouldn't have referred her to him again if she required further surgery. Tempting fate once was enough. Fortunately, she never required any other surgical procedures and died at the age of 82 while tending her flower garden.

As for sending the second patient home with a rigid surgical abdomen and a white count of twenty-four thousand, this is obviously the worst kind of deviation from good medical care that any physician could imagine.

Chapter Twelve

A Matter of Fat

Author's Note:
One of my colleagues, who shall remain anonymous, practicing in a western state, heard through the medical grapevine that I was writing a medical book. He called me and said he had an idea for an interesting article and wondered if I could use it in my book. I thought the idea was good. He supplied all the documentation, I wrote the article, he liked the result, and here is the finished product.

EZ

I was sitting comfortably, half-asleep, waiting for medical rounds to begin. It was already ten after eight and the late stragglers were just dragging in.

"The subject today, gentlemen," the Chief of Medicine said in a loud voice, so the people still chatting would take it as a signal to quiet down, "is 'morbid obesity.'"

I woke up during the few moments that he waited for all the physicians to take their seats.

"The patient was a thirty-year-old female admitted for an intestinal bypass procedure for morbid obesity. She died four days after surgery from a fat embolus."

He presented the essential clinical facts. The radiologist displayed the x-rays that had been done and the pathologist then followed with his findings.

"An interesting secondary finding was a carcinoma of the thyroid," the pathologist said as he concluded. "The clinical chart does not indicate that the thyroid was examined."

I knew very little about intestinal bypass surgery for the treatment of morbid obesity. By definition, the diagnosis is established when the weight is at least one hundred pounds above normal. The operation consisted of bypassing a portion of the small bowel, thereby preventing the body from absorbing as much food. But the operation is controversial. Even though it sounded like a simple procedure, it caused a myriad of serious complications and therefore, was considered experimental. It was performed infrequently, and only in the larger medical centers. I had read briefly that a trial was being conducted in a western university medical center by the National Institutes of Health.

I was shocked to hear that the procedure was being performed in our small community hospital. I was even more astounded to find three more female patients in our medical clinic a few days later, where I was on duty every Monday for 3 months, who had undergone the procedure at our hospital, all by the same surgeon. Upon their discharge from the hospital, they were all sent to the indigent medical clinic for follow-up care. That was enough to make me explode. So what does a good doctor do when he doesn't know what to do? He orders a batch of laboratory tests. And that's exactly what I did. It's like lighting a match in the dark, frequently revealing a path to follow. The patients were advised to return in one week. That gave me enough time to study the type of post-operative problems that could arise in such individuals.

I was in for more shocks. These patients were prone to develop all kinds of serious complications following surgery. I called the medical school library and obtained copies of the major reports written by all the experts throughout the country who had extensive experience with this type of surgery. I was overwhelmed by the dire consequences of this procedure.

Every week I saw more patients sent to the clinic for post-operative care following bypass surgery. Apparently, the surgeon performing this procedure had gone through all the files of obese patients in the clinic. He saw them once in his office, convinced them that surgery would solve their problem permanently, and then dumped them back in the clinic for post-operative care. I understood why he dumped them when I became familiar with all the complications these patients had.

After I collected all the information from the medical school library and made a summary of the involved patients' charts, I wrote the following letter to the Chief of Surgery, Dr. Joseph Donner:

Dr. Joseph Donner
Chief of Surgery
Commonwealth Community Hospital
Centerville, RK 9961082

Dear Dr. Donner,

As you remember, at the last quarterly staff meeting I mentioned the fact that I had seen a patient in the indigent medical clinic who had undergone intestinal bypass surgery for morbid obesity. At that time, I was upset because I felt I should not be required to see a surgical patient who is suffering from iatrogenic disease (physician caused) which is the direct result of a surgical procedure that the operating surgeon has no inclination to follow himself. No surgeon has the right to dump his problems on the medical clinics. Furthermore, I felt that any surgical procedure that appeared to worsen the patient by deliberately creating a malabsorption syndrome with all its dire consequences of liver failure, hypokalemia (low potassium), hypocalcemia (low calcium), chronic diarrhea, hypovitaminosis (low vitamin levels), etc., must be intrinsically wrong.

I therefore retreated to the medical school library for further information regarding this procedure. Important excerpts from the literature follow:

"The patient should be worked up and followed by an internist or an endocrinologist who understands the serious metabolic changes that take place following the intestinal bypass, particularly in relation to the liver changes. It is my firm belief that this operation should not be done by the occasional operator and should be confined to the major centers where all the facilities are available for proper follow-up."—*Payne.*

"This operation in obese patients does cause malabsorption and protein malnutrition with fatty liver (liver degeneration where fat replaces liver cells), and occasionally peripheral neuropathy (degeneration of nerves), and other signs of vitamin deficiency. Since calcium loss may be excessive, the operation should not be used in patients who have abnormal calcium metabolism, or in the presence of any condition that could cause malabsorption, liver disease, or impaired protein metabolism. These patients must be observed closely for signs of liver disease, hypoproteinemia (low protein levels), hypocalcemia, chronic dehydration, formation of renal stones, decalcification of bones, and peripheral neuropathy. Persistent abnormalities may need restoration of intestinal continuity. All operations for treatment of obesity are still under study and their usefulness cannot be stated at this time."—*Mason*.

"It is my opinion that such an operative treatment for obesity is worth considering as a last resort in selected patients if all dietary attempts at weight reduction have failed; the patient and family have been advised of and are willing to accept the potential risks; the patient is emotionally stable, has family support, and agrees to long-term medical observation with careful attention to vitamin and mineral replacement; and there is close cooperation between internist and surgeon who are on the watch for and can promptly correct complications, if and when they occur. Further, long-term follow-up is needed before the final results of such surgery can be fully assessed."—*Frame*

"The mortality of intestinal bypass surgery is about 5% but who would recommend a drug for obesity that was as dangerous as that?"—*Parfitt*

"In contrast, bypass surgery was followed variously by massive fatty changes (of the liver), cholestasis (suppression of the flow of bile), polynuclear inflammatory infiltrates (cells of inflammation), diffuse fibrosis (scarring of the liver), bile duct proliferation, and fatal hepatic necrosis (gangrene of the liver). Morphological changes occurred while liver function tests were still within normal limits. Follow-up biopsy examinations (of the liver) are the only reliable means of judging whether a bypass procedure is causing progressive parenchymal (functioning cells of an organ as compared to the framework of an organ, or stroma) damage. The prevalence of liver damage seems high enough to warrant this recommendation."—*Drenech et al.*

"Each patient must be emotionally well-motivated, neither hostile nor depressed, and must be willing to participate and cooperate in an investigational study."—*Payne et al.*

"It must be emphasized that the bypass operation should not be abused by physicians who select patients who do not meet the rigid indications."—*Payne et al.*

"We have found that 45 patients have suffered 97 complications. In the follow-up period, 36 patients have had to be rehospitalized a total of 69 times. You must be prepared for a long drawn-out period of careful observation."—*Goldfarb.*

"This operation should be limited to patients who are part of a study."—*Scott.*

"If you decide to do this operation, you must have more than one assistant. You need at least two assistants, and preferably three..."—*Ziffren.*

"These operations are dangerous, particularly because of severe respiratory and metabolic problems that arise in the early post-operative days. Every attempt should be made to obtain weight reduction by other means before operation is advised. The average food intake (estimated at 8000 calories per day) indicates the concomitant psychiatric problem. Only large centers are equipped with the necessary means to engage in these procedures."—*Welch.*

Not one of the investigators emphasized the simple fact that this operation causes complications in 100% of the cases.

One of the cases done at this hospital recently, ended at autopsy four days later from a fat embolus. This case was presented at our medical department meeting. (#926948276).

A study of the chart reveals the following:

1. The patient had no prior study of her endocrine status. The levels of calcium, potassium, proteins, lipid profile, or liver studies were not done. The functions of the thyroid, pituitary, or adrenals were not assessed. At autopsy a carcinoma of the thyroid was found. This was not discovered on physical examination before surgery because the thyroid was not examined. No internist saw the patient before surgery. A brief and totally inadequate pulmonary assessment was on the chart. A brief and totally inadequate psychiatric note was also on the chart. This did, however, reveal that the patient suffered from chronic depression caused by the death of a child eight years ago. This is a specific contraindication for surgery, yet she was allowed to undergo this procedure. There was no assessment of her renal status. No bowel x-rays were performed. No skull x-rays were done to rule out a pituitary tumor.

2. Following the surgery, when the patient began to deteriorate clini-

cally, no consultation was obtained until shortly before her death, when it was already too late to do anything.

At autopsy, death was found to be the result of fat emboli. Operative notes list only a nurse as an assistant.

Another patient who had the same procedure done at another hospital in this state, died recently in our hospital and you may also want to see that chart. (#92684292). Death was caused by bowel obstruction with subsequent perforation and peritonitis.

I have studied the chart of J.T., one of the patients I had seen in the medical clinic last week and have the following to report:

The patient was hospitalized recently with a kidney infection. She was hospitalized again three months later with the same problem. There was no consultation with a urologist during either of the two hospitalizations. A few liver studies were done and were abnormal. No thyroid studies were done. The sodium and potassium levels were not obtained before surgery. One fasting blood sugar was done and found to be significantly elevated, but never repeated. There is no mention of the patient being a diabetic, even though this diagnosis was established two years ago. It was also established two years ago, during a hospitalization at this institution, that this patient was suffering from a chronic anxiety state. There is a brief and totally inadequate psychiatric note in the chart. The evaluation of this patient was extremely cursory and not performed to protect the patient.

Four months after surgery, the patient was again hospitalized with a psychiatric diagnosis of depressive neurosis. On physical examination, the liver was found to be enlarged and tender and five centimeters below the right costal (rib) margin. The liver scan was read as "enlarged liver with diminished concentration."

It is distressing to note that the patient was admitted with a urinary tract infection and after a superficial workup, was subjected to intestinal bypass surgery a few days later.

These horrible things are happening here at this hospital, in your department, under your very nose.

Nowhere have I seen statistics proving these patients have a better and longer life following this surgical procedure. In fact, the opposite is true. This is brutalizing surgery.

Because of this, I would like you to review the charts of all the patients who have undergone this procedure at this hospital. I feel that the rigid criteria for the selection of these patients have been totally disregarded, the workup is completely inadequate, and proper post-operative care has been neglected.

When patients like these are dumped on the indigent medical clinic and seen by physicians totally unschooled in the problems presented by intestinal bypass surgery, I believe drastic steps should be taken immediately to prevent this from ever happening again.

After studying the literature, there is no doubt in my mind our community hospital is in no way equipped or staffed to allow this type of surgery to be done. Therefore, I expect you, in your capacity as Chief of Surgery, to immediately stop intestinal bypass procedures from being done at this hospital.

Sincerely,
R.T.L.

After this letter, all hell broke loose. My life was miserable for the next two years. One week after receiving my letter, the Chief of Surgery called me, stating the surgeon in question told him that all the bypass procedures done at our hospital were a part of a government study being conducted in a university medical center in another state.

"Who told you that?" I said.

"Dr. Quarry, who else? The very man you're attacking."

"I find that hard to believe," I said. "Are you going to stop him from doing the surgery?"

"Absolutely not," he said. "This is a legitimate study. He is a qualified surgeon. And the surgery will continue."

"No, it won't," I said. "You must know by now that when I know I'm right, I never give up."

"You're a gadfly, Doctor," he said, "and gadflies are known to get hurt. I know you're a good family physician. All your patients like you. You're well trained and you're conscientious. Why jeopardize your career? Dr. Quarry's planning to hire an attorney and he's undoubtedly going to sue you if you don't drop this matter."

"So it has come to that, *threats*. Well, I'm not going to drop it. I also know he'll never sue me. I can play hardball, too, you know. If I get up on that witness stand and accuse him of murdering that young woman whose chart we reviewed at our medical department meeting, his career in this town will be over and he knows it. In fact, he'll probably land in jail."

I called the Dean of the medical school where the government study was supposedly being done. He was a classmate of mine, a fact Dr. Quarry didn't know.

"I'll call you back within the hour," he said. "Let me do some checking."

One hour later, the Dean was back on the phone.

"He is definitely not a part of the study being carried out in this center," he said. "We have never even heard of this individual."

With a little effort and cooperation from the record room, I was able to locate every chart of every patient that had the operation in our hospital. Dr. Quarry had performed the operation three times more often than the surgeons at the Mayo Clinic, and twice as many times as the surgeons doing the government study.

I imparted this information to the Chief of Surgery.

"I don't care what you find out," he said. "I'm not going to do anything about it and that's final."

"No, it isn't final," I said. "How many deaths are you going to allow?"

"That's the business of the surgical department of this hospital, in case you have forgotten. And I just happen to be the chief of that department, I might add. I am not going to allow a family physician to determine the kind of surgical procedures that will be permitted in this hospital. If you persist in this foolishness, you'll end up losing your privileges here."

"So that's what's bothering you. Instead of worrying about the patients, you're worrying about me usurping your power as chief of the department. Well, you're going to have to bend sooner or later. I hope you'll bend while you still have your head on your shoulders. After all, you're responsible for the level of surgical skills in your department."

The next day as I was finishing rounds, I saw Dave Ringer, the administrator of the hospital coming towards me.

"Can I talk to you?" he said.

"Of course," I said.

"When are you going to stop this vendetta against Dr. Quarry?" he said.

"Who told you it's a vendetta?" I said.

"The grapevine," he said.

"Well, the grapevine is wrong," I said. "I'm doing this because Dr. Quarry is performing a bad procedure in this hospital, one that is experimental, to boot. This should never be allowed in a small community hospital like this. And if the Chief of Surgery had been doing his job properly, we wouldn't even be discussing this problem at this moment."

"You're not in the surgical department," he said. "I'd advise you to keep your nose out of this affair, or otherwise you may be very sorry."

"Well, I've been getting some great words of encouragement lately," I said. "The Chief of Surgery threatened me with the loss of my privileges and he's not even in my department. He said that Dr. Quarry plans to sue me. And now, *you are threatening me. This is going to look great for all of you when we meet in court.*"

He started to walk away, looking disgusted.

"Tell the Chief of Surgery to do his job. When he does, that's when I'll stop my campaign. Remember, I'm a member of the staff here. Anything bad that happens in this hospital reflects on all of us. That's what motivates me, in case you didn't know. Now go do your job and get the Chief of Surgery to do his. Then you won't have to go around threatening people, and we'll all be happy. And while you're at it, brush up on your knowledge of 'Due Process.' It might help you from making yourself look totally ridiculous."

This is certainly not the way to make friends and influence people, I thought to myself. But I'd had enough. I put up with another three months of constant harassment from various surgeons, the administrator, and even several members of the Board of Trustees. Nobody jumped on me from the medical department, because they all recognized that these bypass cases were a sad reflection on the hospital. Things gradually quieted down, however. There was less and less talk, a gradual decrease in the level of harassment, and finally silence regarding the procedure. Dr. Quarry, during that time, performed only one more intestinal bypass and then stopped.

There was no lawsuit. I didn't lose my privileges. And in my heart I knew that I had done the right thing and that was what mattered. After all, that's what I was trained to do.

PATIENT BEWARE—

Two years later, the executive committee, our own elected representatives, gave Dr. Quarry a light reprimand for operating with insufficient reasons on too many patients. Nothing more. That reprimand didn't change his operating methods in any way.

LESSONS TO BE LEARNED

"Obesity is a life-long challenge with no quick or easy fixes." This was the conclusion of an expert government investigative commission as reported recently in the American Medical News. About seventy-five million Americans are overweight. These fat people are not happy being fat. And obesity shortens life in a variety of ways. Furthermore, there is considerable discrimination against fat people in our society that is rarely, if ever, discussed. So when a physician offers a "quick fix," there are going to be many people who will be willing to try it without thinking of the risks involved.

There is a simple lesson here: no experimental surgery of any type should be performed in a small community hospital. The surgery, itself, may be a simple procedure to a well-trained surgeon. However, the after-care could end up being very complicated and require a team effort. A team working together on a daily basis is going to do a better job than a team that is hurriedly and haphazardly thrown together for a procedure once every three months. The hospital administration may be very permissive on questionable surgical procedures because of the high cash flow they generate.

Recently, hospitals have turned to weight programs involving liquid protein diets. The charge for one year has been approximately three thousand dollars. Fortunately, because of the recession and the fact that they are not cost-effective, these programs are gradually being terminated. There is also a high incidence of gall bladder disease associated with these liquid protein diet programs.

The sad truth, unfortunately, is that we don't have any easy answers regarding obesity. Until we do, we will have to rely on a restricted diet, exercise, and a life-long commitment to behavior modification.

PATIENT BEWARE—

Patients should not undergo experimental procedures without first consulting their own physicians.

Chapter Thirteen

The Prostate, the Platelet, and the Pulmonary Shadow

Gustave Rinder was a big, affable individual. He had an aura about him that immediately aroused everybody's attention in the waiting room. Actually, it wasn't his size, or the bushy mustache, or the kindly look on his face, that had everybody glancing his way. It was the smell of manure and hay that traveled with him wherever he went. He was a cattle farmer, one of a dying breed in Connecticut. He raised polled Herefords, and his herd was a beautiful sight as they grazed on the hills of his farm only a few miles from my office.

I'd recognize the smell the minute Gus walked into my office, having raised Herefords and Quarter horses myself.

"It's a sorry day, Doctor," he said, smoothing down his mustache with the fingers of his right hand, "when a man loses the ability to take a decent piss, and I might add, the pleasure of doing so."

"Is that your problem, Gus, or is that just your philosophical comment on the aging process in man, generally speaking?"

"No, unfortunately, that's my problem," Gus said. "It's been getting worse every day now for the past six months."

"Do you have to get up at night to pass your water?"

"I might as well sleep in the bathroom," he said. "Every two hours, I'm up."

After his examination, I checked the necessary laboratory work and then came back to his room.

He looked at me like a big sad bear from a Walt Disney movie.

"Well, Doctor, give me the bad news," he said.

"You have an enlarged prostate, Gus, and it's blocking the flow of urine from your bladder."

"It's not cancer, is it?"

"It doesn't feel like cancer, Gus, but we won't know for sure until we do more tests and perform a biopsy."

"So what do you suggest I do about it?" he said.

"If you continue to delay surgery, eventually the prostate will block the flow completely and your surgery will then have to be done on an emergency basis. But if you decide on surgery now, I'll arrange for you to see a urologist, a specialist in this field. He'll have you admitted to the hospital and under anesthesia, insert a tube into your penis and cut out the parts of the prostate that are blocking the flow of urine. This procedure is called a TURP, or a transurethral resection of the prostate. Probably many of your friends have already had it done."

"Yes, they have," he said. "And they all seem to be doing fairly well."

"Well, generally that's true, but with any type of surgery you can always run into various kinds of problems, too," I said.

"Like what?" he said.

"The urologist will go over all the complications that can develop, Gus, but I can tell you it's a relatively safe procedure. According to the statistics, about 10-15% of the men complain of impotence after surgery and a small number have trouble controlling their urination."

"That sounds just wonderful to look forward to, Doctor," Gus said.

Gus was admitted the following week. The surgery itself, was uneventful, but he wouldn't stop bleeding. At first, there was just a trickle with a few clots. This amount of bleeding is not unusual with this procedure. But instead of slowing down within the next few days, the bleeding worsened.

Bleeding is controlled naturally in the body by minute circular or oval particles in the blood called platelets, along with other blood factors manufactured by the liver. Before surgery, all patients undergo a variety of blood tests, one of them being an actual count of these particles. The normal count is 250,000 to 400,000 per cubic millimeter of blood.

Before surgery, Gus's platelet count was normal. Within three days after surgery, his count dropped to 40,000 and he began to hemorrhage.

We pumped unit after unit of packed red cells, whole blood, and platelets into him trying to keep up with his constant hemorrhaging. The hematologist we called in as a consultant ordered massive doses of cortisone intravenously. After one week of flirting with death, Gus gradually stopped bleeding. His platelet count rose to 60,000 and stabilized at that level. Two weeks after surgery, he was finally discharged.

"You're a mighty lucky manure kicker, Gus," I said.

"Thanks to you, the surgeon, and that other doctor you called in. I don't even know his name. How many units of blood did you give me, anyway?"

"You had about forty units of blood, Gus," I said, "plus many units of platelets. I lost count, actually."

"Do you think I'd make it if I ever had to have another operation?"

"The chances are very good that you would bleed to death. Even now, your platelet count is only 60,000, while the normal count is 250,000 to 400,000. We'll keep you on Prednisone and hope that your count gradually returns to normal. In the meantime, be careful what you do. If you're involved in an accident and you get cut, we may not be able to control any bleeding that may occur. And remember, don't take any aspirin."

Over the next three months, the platelet count remained stable at 60,000. There was no further bleeding. I gradually weaned him off his Prednisone.

"There is one thing I want to warn you about, Gus," I said, during one of his examinations.

"What's that?" he said.

"That little shadow about the size of a dime you have on your chest x-ray in the upper lobe of your right lung," I said.

"You told me about that a long time ago," he said.

"That shadow hasn't changed in the past ten years, Gus. But I'm afraid that if you ever develop a severe upper respiratory infection and I don't happen to be around, whoever sees you in the emergency room or in one of those walk-in centers will order a chest x-ray. When they see that shadow, they'll immediately suspect cancer of the lung in a man your age. You'll be referred to a chest surgeon, and more than likely, he'll suggest surgery. And if you do get operated on, you'll die from exsanguination."

"What's that?" he said.

"Loss of blood," I said.

Gus had no further problems. Periodically, he would come in for a routine blood count. The platelet count continued to hold steady around 60,000. He had no bleeding episodes.

About six months later, I went on my regular summer vacation to Nova Scotia. Dr. Sam Cutler covered for me while I was gone. He left on his vacation the day I got back, so I didn't have a chance to talk to him about any of the problems that had come up in my absence.

That afternoon, I received a call from a hematologist in a nearby city.

"Your patient, Gus Rinder, is scheduled for surgery tomorrow. Dr. Harry Townsend asked me to do the presurgical exam. What can you tell me about him?"

Dr. Harry Townsend was notorious for doing unnecessary surgery.

"What's the procedure?" I asked, fearing the worst.

"Harry is going to do a right upper lobectomy for carcinoma of the lung."

"You have to stop him," I said.

"What?" the internist said. "Trying to stop Harry from doing surgery is like trying to stop an avalanche."

"You can't let Harry do that surgery," I said. "He's going to kill that old man."

"What makes you say that?" he said.

I told him about the problems Gus had after his transurethral resection of the prostate.

"Furthermore," I said, "that lesion in his right upper lobe is benign. I've got chest films dating back ten years showing no change in its size or appearance. If Harry operates on that patient, you're going to be faced with a patient who exsanguinates. There is absolutely no doubt in my mind about the outcome."

"Do you know Harry Townsend?" the internist said.

"Yes, unfortunately, I do," I said.

"Then you know that my chances of stopping Harry from operating are just about zero."

"You still have to do it," I said.

"I'll try," he said. There was no conviction in his voice.

Three days later, I saw Gus Rinder's obituary in the paper. I called the internist immediately.

"You were right," he said.

"Exactly what happened?"

"Mr. Rinder died from exsanguination," he said, "just as you predicted. The platelets all but disappeared. We pumped unit after unit into him but he just kept on hemorrhaging."

"And the chest lesion?"

"The path report said it was benign."

Dr. Harry Townsend got thirty-five hundred dollars for killing Gus Rinder. Gus's children were all grateful for everything he did for their father. One year later, Dr. Harry Townsend was elected president of his medical society. A year after that, he received a special commendation for service to the community. There has been no change in his operating methods.

LESSONS TO BE LEARNED

Here is a poor, elderly patient with a benign chest lesion and a low platelet count falling into the hands of an unscrupulous surgeon. And the patient had been warned in advance. So why did he submit? The surgeon is a great persuader. He goes through the charade of calling in a hematologist when he happens to discover the platelet abnormality on routine pre-operative blood work. But does he heed the hematologist's warning about the near exsanguination of this patient during previous surgery? Of course not. Does he sound like some previous surgeons we met before? This surgeon was trained to operate and by God he's going to operate no matter what the consequences. Are there many surgeons like this? Thank God they're in the minority, but there are still too many of them around.

I will not discuss in depth the monetary rewards for surgical intervention compared to the total lack of compensation for careful observation of certain conditions over a period of time. Remember ten years had elapsed since we first discovered this lesion in his chest and it hadn't changed in all that length of time. There is no doubt that surgeons have always been handsomely rewarded for their operative procedures, while primary physicians continue to be the unsung heroes of medicine. The surgeons are the darlings of all hospital administrators because of the great sums of money surgery brings to their institutions.

There has always been a great disparity between compensation of primary physicians compared to surgeons. And I believe this disparity seduces some of the surgeons to be rather liberal in their approach to operative procedures versus medical treatment of many problems seen in medicine today.

Some people may think my impression is just a "sour grapes"

reaction. Let them think as they please. But let me cite an example of this inequality. Back in 1955 when I first entered private practice, an insurance plan offered by Blue Shield paid $5.00 a day starting on the third day of hospitalization for a myocardial infraction or any other serious problem requiring intensive medical care. This plan paid a total of $20.00 for the first week of such care. This same plan paid a surgeon $20.00 for a 5 minute surgical procedure on an ingrown toenail. That disparity between medical care and surgery still exists today, and is now even worse. Is it any wonder that young doctors are refusing to go into primary care?

Are some surgeons motivated by monetary compensation and even greed? Of course. That has been well documented in our society. They are just like any other human beings. Fortunately, these doctors are in the minority.

Chapter Fourteen

The Entangled Tube

Martha Talbot was still a striking woman even though she was eighty years old. We called her a variety of names in the office: "Lady of the Lake," (because she lived near a lake), "The Queen Mother," (because of her regal manner), and "Mrs. Blue Eyes," (because of the beautiful contrast of her blue eyes and white hair).

She suffered from hypertension and hardening of the arteries in her lower extremities. She had considerable pain when she tried to walk more than fifty feet.

On her regular visits every three months, I would ask her if she could still walk to her mailbox by the road.

"I just about make it," she'd say, her head bobbing a little from the tremor she had. "I'm the only one in the neighborhood with a lawn chair by my mailbox in the middle of winter, where I have to sit for five minutes before I can walk back to the house."

Her husband, Charles, who had died ten years before, used to play the oboe for the Boston Symphony Orchestra. Martha had never given up her love of classical music, so when she came in, she would update my appointment book with the "dates of all the important events like symphony concerts and operas that really mattered in a person's life."

She had refused any surgery on her legs to improve her circulation. She had no pulses in her feet or in the femoral arteries in her groins.

"We'll just let nature take its course," she said, quietly but firmly. "After all, I have already overstayed my journey on this planet and besides, Charles is waiting for me with his oboe. Have you heard the beautiful oboe solo in the Gypsy Baron Overture, Doctor?"

The day I admitted her to the hospital, however, she had a new complaint.

"Every time I try to do anything, I get this severe pain in the center of my chest, just as if an elephant had decided to sit on it."

She held her clenched fist against her chest.

"It seems to extend into my left arm," she said, "and all the way up into my jaw. Even my false teeth seem to ache."

She smiled weakly.

"And you drove here by yourself?" I said.

"Of course," she said.

"And how long have you been having these pains?" I said.

"About a week," she said. "I suppose I should have called you but..."

"Yes, Martha," I said. "I already know your philosophy regarding such matters. You were going to let nature take its course."

"Exactly," she said. "So I waited until my regular appointment."

I took her hand.

"Thirty years in practice, Martha," I said, "and you women haven't driven me out of my mind, yet. That's not the world's record but it's getting there."

An EKG did not reveal the typical changes of a myocardial infarction, (heart attack), but did show a marked depression of her ST segment, indicating a severe coronary artery insufficiency.

I arranged for her admission to the Intensive Coronary Care Unit and called in a cardiologist as a consultant. The diagnosis was unstable angina, and in such cases the patient is frequently in imminent danger of a myocardial infarction.

Her unstable angina, however, subsided rather quickly over the next few days as soon as she was given nitroglycerin intravenously. This medication dilates the coronary arteries and improves the circulation.

She refused to have anything else done.

"Now that I no longer have to put up with that insufferable

pain...," she said, pausing and smiling.

"We'll let nature take its course," I finished the sentence for her.

"Exactly," she said. "You're getting to know my every thought, Doctor."

She dropped her eyes coquettishly.

"Well, almost every thought," she added.

Nature did take its course. On the day she was scheduled for discharge, she suddenly developed rectal bleeding.

"Have you had any bleeding like this before, Martha?" I said.

"I have to confess, Doctor, that I haven't been completely honest with you. Please don't scold me. The truth is, I've had some rectal bleeding off and on for the past month."

"You are a naughty woman, Martha," I said. "I can't do my job properly unless you tell me everything."

"Well, that's everything," she said. "Now what?"

"Now, we have to scope you, Martha, and see where that bleeding is coming from."

"Oh dear," she said. "I was afraid you were going to say that. Couldn't it be just hemorrhoids?"

"Yes, it could," I said. "But your rectal exam on admission to the hospital was unremarkable and at your age, we worry about something more devastating."

"You mean what you doctors call the 'Big C?'" she said.

"Yes," I said.

"Well, let's get it over with, Doctor," she said. "I'm not going to complain."

I called in a surgeon who performed a colonoscopy on her the next day. The pathology report proved it was the "Big C." Fortunately, the cancer was located in the ascending colon, which is on the right side of the abdominal cavity, so that a primary resection could be performed without a colostomy. A cancer in this area rarely gives early symptoms because the contents of the bowel are in a liquid state and obstruction doesn't occur early in the disease.

"You know that I couldn't tolerate a colostomy, Doctor," Martha said, sitting up primly in her bed. "Never, never, never. I would just have to..."

"Let nature take its course," I said.

"Exactly," she said.

"Martha," I said, "I've known you for over twenty-five years, and I would be willing to bet that you could tolerate anything that you had to tolerate."

"Well, I suppose so, if I really had to," she said.

She had her surgery and in spite of her coronary artery insufficiency and the lack of circulation in her lower extremities, her post-operative progress was excellent. On the third day after her surgery, however, her belly began to bloat. She developed a "paralytic ileus," a condition in which all contractions of the bowel cease and the belly begins to bloat with gas, a situation not uncommon following intestinal surgery in the elderly.

"Now what?" she said, her hands holding onto her big, distended belly.

"Now, we have to insert a gastric tube through your nose down to your stomach and apply some suction. While we are getting rid of your bloated belly, we'll continue to give you intravenous fluids just as we have been doing for the last few days since your surgery."

"And I thought I'd be eating by now," she said.

"You will in a few days," I said. "As soon as your belly goes down and your intestines decide to start working again."

"Well, let's get on with it," she said.

Within three days, her belly was completely down and I could hear the faint sounds of peristalsis beginning.

"Now you should make rapid progress and get out of here in a few more days," I said. "As soon as you start passing gas."

"What a horrible expression," she said.

"Even the Queen Mother passes gas," I said.

"I suppose so, but discretely, and in a royal manner, I'm sure."

When the surgeon attempted to pull out the gastric tube the next day, it appeared to be stuck. By x-ray we could see that the tube had coiled upon itself, forming a loose knot.

"That's odd," I said to the surgeon. "I've never seen that happen before."

"Neither have I," the surgeon said. "It's been reported in the literature, however."

"What are you planning to do about it? Are you going to scope her?"

"No, not yet. I hate to subject her to a gastroscopy after all she's been through. I'll play around with it for a day or so and see if I can untangle it. She is doing well and there's no hurry."

Two days later, I saw the surgeon in the hallway. He was smiling.

"I managed to get that damn tube out without scoping her," he said. "I tugged and tugged every day, gently of course, and it finally slipped out."

"Was it still coiled up in a knot," I said.

"Yes, it was, but I was happy to see it come out."

Twenty-four hours later, Martha spiked a fever to 105 degrees. We placed a cooling blanket on her and started her on broad-range antibiotics.

"Why do you think she spiked this fever all of a sudden when she had been doing so well?" I asked the surgeon.

"Well, you know that aspiration pneumonia is a common problem in elderly patients post-operatively. They have such a poor gag reflex that some of their saliva slips down into their lungs. A pulmonary embolus from a deep thrombophlebitis in her lower extremities is another possibility."

But Martha didn't have any inflammation or pains in her legs. She didn't have stabbing pains in her chest and she wasn't spitting up blood.

But she did complain of severe pain in the right upper quadrant of her abdomen. On palpation, she had marked spasm with rebound pain.

"Martha didn't have any gall stones, did she, when you explored her abdomen at surgery?" I asked the surgeon when I saw him later that day.

"No, her gall bladder was normal."

"How about a liver abscess?" I said.

"That's a good possibility," he said.

Martha's condition deteriorated rapidly. Her temperature hovered around 105 degrees continuously. She slipped quietly into a coma and died on her fifth post-operative day.

At autopsy, for which I had permission from Martha's son, while the surgeon maintained a discrete silence, the pathologist found a four inch linear tear in the esophagus where it joined the stomach. Apparently, the entangled gastric tube hadn't come out as easily as the surgeon had thought.

I called Martha's son in Maine and told him what had happened.

He thanked me for being so honest with him.

As he hung up, I heard him starting to cry.

The surgeon was a good doctor and he felt terrible. I knew he would never repeat that mistake.

LESSONS TO BE LEARNED

There are several interesting points to discuss here. For unstable angina, intravenous nitroglycerin quickly became the drug of choice in coronary intensive care units because of its unique ability to relax the vascular musculature in the coronary arteries and throughout the body. The cardiologists quickly restricted its use to their specialty. Only a cardiologist should be allowed to monitor the administration of this drug, they chorused throughout the nation, because of the possibility of severe hypotension (the collapse of normal blood pressure) in inexperienced hands, with subsequent damage to the kidneys, brain, heart, and liver.

The patients ended up on a continuous intravenous drip of nitroglycerin for many days as the cardiologists *carefully* monitored its administration. Then lo and behold, a study was done that proved the efficacy of continued intravenous nitroglycerin lasted only about 24 hours and the patient quickly developed tolerance to the drug soon thereafter. So a drug had been administered intravenously for several days and restricted to careful monitoring by cardiologists during that time, exposing the patient to complete collapse of his blood pressure when it should have been stopped as tolerance developed.

The amazing thing about nitroglycerin is that when I entered clinical practice in 1955, it was considered malpractice to give this drug to a patient with an acute coronary. But this is not the first time the medical profession has done a complete about-face and it isn't the last.

Martha Talbot was willing to discuss her angina but concealed the fact that she had intermittent rectal bleeding for about a month. This isn't an uncommon occurrence in medical practice. Fear is the culprit that blinds the patient to the true nature of the problem.

After undergoing major surgery successfully at her advanced age, she was unfortunate enough to develop a paralytic ileus. This usually is a temporary problem. The gastric tube is inserted and attached to suction and the bowel begins its normal peristaltic action within a few days, but not always. The gastric tube coiling upon itself and forming a knot was an unusual event. The method chosen by the surgeon, consisting of gentle tugging, was obviously the wrong one.

The surgeon was an expert endoscopist. He could have easily inserted a gastroscope and uncoiled the tube. Occasionally, this method is also unsuccessful. The tube, then, can be cut into small sections and removed or allowed to pass through the intestinal tract normally.

The surgeon, unfortunately, opted for tugging on the tube, tearing the esophagus in the process, which led quickly and unalterably to the patient's death.

Chapter Fifteen

A Short Journey

*L*ydia Classon looked directly at me.

"I've decided that I don't want to live anymore," she said, coolly. "I didn't come to this conclusion lightly. You know me better than that, Doctor, so I don't want you to try to talk me out of it."

Her husband, Clyde, was sitting next to her, looking very uncomfortable. He couldn't keep his legs still.

"Did anything happen recently to make you come to this conclusion?" I said.

"No, I don't believe anything in particular happened to make me decide that this is what I should do. You've been treating me for depression for the last twenty years, and I have to admit that sometimes I have felt pretty good. But other times I feel really bad. I just came to the realization that it's senseless to continue this way, overwhelming everybody with my miseries. Since my menopause, I've been much worse, you know that, Doctor."

"I suppose you've spoken to your husband about your intentions," I said.

"Yes, I have," she said. "He told me he wouldn't try to stop me. But at the same time, he asked me to see you one last time before I did anything."

"Well, now that you're here, why don't you give me one more chance to see if I can change your mind," I said.

"No," she said. "If I thought it would help, I'd do what you suggest. But deep in my heart, I know that it would be useless."

"I don't want to bother you by begging for your life, Lydia," I said, "but after you're gone, I'll be the one left behind with your husband and children, wondering the big question?"

"What big question?" she said.

"The question of whether we did all we could to save you, if not for yourself, then at least for your family's sake. Just let me put you in the hospital for one week, Lydia, and I promise you I'll never bother you like this again."

"Why don't you do what the Doctor suggests, Lydia?" Clyde said. "It certainly won't hurt you to give him one final chance to rid you of that depression."

"You know it's useless, dear. We've gone over this many times before. You see, don't you, that I want to set you and our two children free. I've had everybody chained to me for much too long."

"One more time," her husband said. "And like the Doctor said, I'll never bother you again about this problem, either."

Lydia looked at me, then at Clyde, then back at me, almost in exasperation. She finally shrugged her shoulders and threw up her hands in resignation.

"All right, Doctor, I'll give you three days to see if you can change my mind. After that, I don't want either one of you to bother me about this ever again. I don't want to appear ungrateful, Doctor. You've kept me going for the last twenty years. But now it's over."

"Fair enough, Lydia. You can go straight to the hospital from here. I'll call them immediately and leave some orders to make you comfortable. I'll admit you on the medical floor, just as I've done before."

"I have to warn you, Doctor, that I may change my mind on the way to the hospital and come right back home."

"You aren't a prisoner, Lydia. You have to do this of your own free will."

As soon as they left, I called the admitting office and left the orders. I told them to call me as soon as she arrived there.

The rest of the afternoon was a madhouse. I didn't have a moment to myself until we were ready to quit at five o'clock. Since I hadn't heard from the hospital in the last three hours, I assumed that Lydia had changed her mind and decided to go home. I knew her husband would call me if he needed me.

I made three house calls. I then went to the convalescent hospital to see three more patients and finally dragged my weary body home exhausted.

The next day, while I was making rounds on the various floors of the hospital, all the nurses were talking about the patient who had run out in front of the ambulance. Apparently she had smashed all the bones in her lower extremities, her arms and her pelvis, but survived.

I didn't realize they were talking about Lydia Classon until I went to the emergency room to see a patient with pneumonia.

"Your patient certainly made quite a stir yesterday, Doctor," the nursing supervisor said.

"Which patient do you mean?" I said.

None of the floor nurses had mentioned any disturbance caused by any of my patients.

"Lydia Classon," she said.

"What happened?" I said, surprised.

"She came to the emergency room and the crisis worker had her admitted to Dr. Benson's service immediately. When the crisis worker stepped out of the examining room for a moment, Mrs. Classon walked calmly out of the E.R. and stepped directly in the path of an ambulance that was taking off for an emergency."

"So that's what happened to her," I said.

I then told the nursing supervisor that I had made arrangements for Lydia's admission and had assumed she never got to the hospital because nobody called me.

"The crisis worker took a lot upon herself," I said, "to send my patient to the psychiatric wing on Dr. Benson's service. She didn't bother to call me. Didn't she realize that the patient could interpret this as abandonment and also come to the conclusion that I was trying to trick her and have her committed?"

"I guess she didn't think about that," the nursing supervisor said.

"What makes a twenty-four year old crisis worker feel she knows more about handling a suicidal patient whom she had never seen before, than a doctor who's been taking care of that patient for the last twenty-five years?"

"She knows you're not a psychiatrist."

"Yes, but Lydia Classon was my patient and I didn't send her to a twenty-four year old crisis worker for consultation. This little mistake will probably cost the hospital a considerable amount of money if somebody gets around to filing a lawsuit."

Later I spoke to Lydia's husband and found out that it was he who had encouraged the crisis worker to admit his wife on the psychiatric wing because he planned to have her committed to prevent her from committing suicide. He apologized for not mentioning it to me.

Lydia went through six months of convalescence while all her bones healed. During that period of time, she appeared to have overcome her depression and never spoke about her attempt at suicide. She was determined to get well. She faithfully did all the exercises she was taught in physiotherapy and made great strides to full recovery. She refused to see me or a psychiatrist during the entire six months of her convalescence, telling her husband that she now had an entirely different attitude and outlook on life.

"What a fool I've been," she said repeatedly to all her friends.

During that time, it was rumored, but never verified, that a suit had been filed against the hospital.

"That will pay for a nice little journey anywhere in the world," one of the hospital nurses was heard to say.

Lydia was finally discharged from the orthopedic surgeon's care and made an appointment to see me in the office. By then, I was beginning to think that all of us had been victimized in one way or another.

"I've been following your case very closely, Lydia. Dr. Fowler, the orthopedic surgeon, told me that you were a model patient and that was why you were able to make such a remarkable recovery. Furthermore, he told me that you didn't suffer from any depression during that entire period of time. Do you think that we have stumbled on a new way to solve depression by having patients leap in front of an ambulance?"

"I wouldn't want to go through that again," she said. "Broken bones are much worse than electric shock therapy, I'm sure. I really don't know what really happened. I just made up my mind that I had to get better and be totally independent again. My husband and my two children have been a great help to me while I was recovering from those injuries. I know they really love me and that helped a lot."

"You certainly demonstrated to everybody just how strong you really are, Lydia," I said. "You should be proud of yourself."

"The real reason for coming in to see you, Doctor, is to tell you how thankful I am for all the years you have taken care of me. And to tell you, too, how sorry I am for having been such a big burden to you and everybody else. You were always there when I needed you."

"Thank you, Lydia, for coming in to tell me that. You were never a burden. It's amazing how just a few words can make a person feel good. So few patients take the time out to do the very thing you're doing. You know doctors need a little boost themselves, now and then."

I followed her to the door.

"What are your immediate plans, Lydia?"

"I've been planning a short trip now for a long time, in fact, for the past six months. Now that I'm back in shape again, I think I deserve it, don't you, Doctor, after all I've been through?"

"Yes, I do. I know that you'll enjoy your journey no matter where you go, Lydia. You're a remarkable woman. Let me know if you need me in any way. You know that I'm always here to help you. And please say hello to your husband for me, won't you?"

"He's going bowling tonight while I put the finishing touches to my plans."

She gave me a peck on the cheek and left.

She was in a remarkably good mood. I hadn't seen her like this in years. I had a difficult time understanding how she managed to get through several bone operations, extended physiotherapy, with all the misery that accompanies multiple fractures, and still look this well.

What metabolic changes took place in her body and brain to make her depression vanish? Medicine is fascinating and there is so much we don't understand, I thought to myself as I watched her get into her car. Is her depression really gone or is she just acting out a part?

That evening, while her husband was bowling, she doused her bedroom with ten gallons of gasoline, climbed into bed with her cat, and lit a match. She finally took the short journey that she had been planning for the past six months.

LESSONS TO BE LEARNED

Lydia Classon was obviously deeply depressed and suicidal. She had seen several different psychiatrists over the years and had even gone through EST (electroshock therapy). When she appeared improved in between her periods of depression, I couldn't really ascertain whether she was truly better or was just playing the part of a healthy patient. I always had the feeling she was just fooling us and getting some kind of strange enjoyment out of this subterfuge. It almost seemed we were dealing with two distinct personalities, one depressed and the other happy and normal. Whatever it was, she certainly got a lot of attention from her family and her doctors.

The crisis worker, by interfering with the admission process and not bothering to call me, actually precipitated the suicidal attempt. I had promised Lydia that she would be admitted on a regular medical floor, which I had done many times before, much to the dismay of the chief of medicine. Lydia had told me a long time ago that she didn't want to be on the same floor with "all those crazy people." Actually, the young drug addicts were the ones that seemed to bother her the most. When the crisis worker switched her to the psychiatric wing without calling me first, Lydia interpreted this change as a trick to get her committed to the state hospital. She concluded that not only was I involved in this deception, but also that I had abandoned her by doing so. She suspected that her husband was behind the whole affair and had engineered the entire conspiracy.

There was no doubt that she had been suicidal for a long time as she switched back and forth between her depressed and happy personalities. But in the past, she had always been willing to undergo further treatment to see if we could change the course she had plotted for herself. And she always responded well to treatment with her old happy self emerging from the shadowy prison of her mind. It appeared there was a constant battle between her two selves.

The amazing part of this tragedy was that she waited until she had fully recovered from her previous attempt before she decided to go on this short journey.

The lesson here is that once the physician and his depressed patient decide on a plan of treatment, any third person who interferes and forces a change in the plans, well intentioned or not, may precipitate disaster. The patient's interpretation of this sudden change may be far different than the one intended, as demonstrated in this episode of the young crisis worker who thought she was helping.

Chapter Sixteen

A Brief Check-up

"*H*ello, Sally," I said, as I entered the examining room with my nurse. "What can I do for you? You appear to be in excellent health."

She was a pretty, dark-haired woman of about forty with bewitching dimples that made her look sweet and innocent.

"I just dropped in to have my blood pressure checked, Doctor, and you know, my heart and lungs. I haven't had a check-up in over a year."

I met Sally and her husband at the opera a few years before. They lived a few miles down the road in Farmington. Her husband was a top executive in one of the big insurance companies in Hartford.

"But you're feeling well?" I asked, taking her blood pressure.

"Oh, yes, very well," she said smiling. "I play tennis three times a week, swim frequently, work out in a body shop, play golf in the summer, you know, all the things a yuppie is supposed to do."

She didn't ask me what her blood pressure was. I examined her heart and lungs and then her throat and ears.

"Is there anything that you're particularly worried about or that you'd like me to examine. A brief exam is really inadequate unless it's for a follow-up."

I knew she went to a gynecologist for her pap smears.

"No, nothing in particular," she said.

I put my fingers on her thyroid and asked her to swallow. As her thyroid slid up under my fingers, I felt a distinct lump in the right lobe of the gland.

I sat down at the small desk next to the examining table and started to write my notes.

"How's Richard doing?" I asked.

"Oh, he's fine," she said. "He's under a lot of stress, of course, at work, but as long as he has his two martinis every evening he doesn't complain."

She got off the examining table and took a few steps towards the door.

"Are you finished?" she said, her eyes wide open, sweet and innocent. "I suppose you didn't find anything that would make me worry?"

"Did you expect me to find anything, Sally?"

"No, not really. I feel great. Just a little check-up, that's all I wanted."

"I suppose you know that you have a lump in the right lobe of your thyroid," I said.

"Yes, I do," she said. "I found it last week. I was standing in front of the mirror and happened to swallow and I saw a small lump move up and down in the front of my neck. It scared the hell out of me."

"Why didn't you tell me?"

"I wanted to see if you'd find it," she said.

"You know, Sally, this isn't a game that you play with your doctor. You're supposed to tell me everything that's bothering you. We should be working as a team."

"Well, if you missed it, I was going to see my surgeon, anyway."

"Now that we know why you're here—because of the lump in your thyroid—tell me, have you had any radiation to your neck or face in the past?"

"Yes," she said, "I had some acne when I was growing up and I had a course of radiation. Why, is that significant?"

"Yes, it is. There is a higher incidence of adenomas, lumps in the thyroid, in people who had previous radiation. There is also a higher incidence of thyroid cancer. However, the vast majority of thyroid lumps are simple, benign adenomas. I suppose you already have decided on a course of action. What would you like me to do?"

"Call Dr. Cabot for me, will you, Doctor?" she said. "I know that he'll want to take it out right away."

"Before you rush off to surgery, Sally, we should do some thyroid studies. Dr. Cabot will want this basic blood work when you see him."

"Dr. Cabot is one of my father's old friends, Doctor. I'm sure he'll do everything that has to be done. I'd be very happy if you just set up that appointment for me. Make it for tomorrow, please. I don't want to wait another day."

I made the appointment for Sally. Dr. Cabot ordered the appropriate tests including blood work and a radioactive scan and uptake. The following week he excised the mass. The pathology report indicated the lump was a benign adenoma, a gland-like growth.

I didn't see Sally for about a year. She called for another appointment.

It was déjà vu as my nurse and I entered the examining room. There was the same sweet, innocent-looking Sally showing us her dimples.

"Hello, Sally. I haven't seen you and Richard at the opera lately."

"We didn't renew our tickets this year, Doctor. We're really too busy. There just isn't enough time in the day to do all the things we'd like to do. I don't even have time to smell the flowers. You know I'm president of the Women's Club this year and every day is simply a whirlwind. I just dropped in for a brief check-up, you know, my heart and lungs and blood pressure and so forth. I really don't have time for a complete physical examination."

"Dr. Cabot did a great job excising that adenoma," I said. "The scar is barely visible. I hope you're taking your thyroid medication."

"Dr. Cabot didn't give me any thyroid medication. He said I don't need anything and I've been feeling well."

I went through the brief routine as before. She again didn't bother to ask me what her blood pressure was.

"I suppose you've had your breasts checked, your abdomen, and everything else," I said.

"Oh my, yes," she said. "My gynecologist, Bill Clapper, attends to all those parts. He even checks my cholesterol."

She laughed.

"But I think everybody should have a family doctor and that's why I'm here for my annual check-up."

"You can hardly call this a check-up, Sally," I said.

"I don't have time for anything more extensive, Doctor," she said smiling, dimples showing.

I put my fingers on her thyroid and asked her to swallow. As the thyroid slid up and down, I felt a small lump in the *left* lobe of her thyroid.

I sat down at the desk to write my notes.

"I suppose you already know you have a lump on the other side of your thyroid."

"Yes, I do," she said. "Call Dr. Cabot for me, like a dear, won't you? Next Wednesday is open for me. He can take the lump out then."

"This time," I said, "make sure he doesn't forget to put you on thyroid medication. That will suppress your thyroid from developing new adenomas."

"I'll leave that up to Dr. Cabot. You know he's an old family friend. He's like a father to me. Such a glorious man."

Another appointment was made for Sally to see Dr. Cabot. After appropriate tests, which he outlined in his report to me, he excised the mass in the left lobe of the thyroid. Again the pathology report revealed the lump to be a benign adenoma

I didn't see Sally for another year and suddenly there she was sitting in the examining room smiling at me with her sweet, little-girl innocence, her dimples deeper then ever. She appeared to have gained some weight.

Like Yogi, the great philosopher, once said when breaking out of his state of meditation, it was déjà vu all over again.

On this third visit, I found another lump in her thyroid, this time in the isthmus.

She admitted Dr. Cabot hadn't prescribed any thyroid medication and that she was gaining weight.

"I probably wouldn't have taken it if he had," she said, with her girlish giggle. "I feel so great and I'm too busy to fuss with medicine, especially if I don't need it. Anyway, one of my neighbors told me thyroid tablets made her practically jump out of her skin. I'm already functioning at full-speed-ahead and I don't need anything like that."

Dr. Cabot again performed the surgery. The pathology report

revealed papillary carcinoma This time he placed Sally on thyroid replacement therapy. She found time every day to take her medication. She even found time to "smell the flowers."

LESSONS TO BE LEARNED

Thyroid adenomas are new growths of gland-like tissue enclosed in a fibrous capsule. Most are found as solitary nodules and usually are asymptomatic. Occasionally, however, they may cause hoarseness, dysphagia (difficulty swallowing), or even pain, depending on the location. They are more common in women and are present in about 2% of the population. They can be present for long periods of time without any danger to the patient.

The problem for the clinician, of course, is to determine if the nodule is benign or malignant. A history of prior radiation to the area will increase the chance of malignancy.

These adenomas are usually found in otherwise normal thyroids. What increases the importance of the problem is that laboratory tests, radioisotope scanning and uptake, along with clinical examination commonly do not reveal the possibility of malignancy. If there is sudden growth or enlargement of the adjacent lymph nodes, the chances of malignancy are much greater. Children and men with solitary nodules are more likely to have carcinoma than women.

Thyroid medication is used to suppress the development of nodules. They can be followed for long periods of time if no changes in their characteristics are found. Patients who undergo surgery for benign adenomas should be placed on thyroid replacement therapy permanently.

Many of the tumors are dependent on TSH (thyroid stimulating hormone) secreted by the pituitary. By placing the patient on thyroid replacement therapy, the TSH is suppressed and the patient usually lives out her life normally.

The problem as illustrated by Sally is the fragmentation of her examination and treatment. She has divided herself among a family physician, a gynecologist, and a surgeon. She has made herself the grand director of her health. She makes all the decisions about what parts of her anatomy will be examined and what medications will be taken. Furthermore, she indulges in a game to see if the physician can find out what she already knows. This type of patient is no help to the physician when the history is taken.

This isn't teamwork. Teamwork, as everybody knows, requires a team captain and cooperation between all members of the team. Without a captain the team will flounder and there will be chaos and blunders without end. One of the problems of medicine today is that patients have been allowed to go to super-specialists without specific advice from a generalist such as an internist or family physician. The costs of such unrestricted, undirected medical care are prohibitive.

For example, let's see what happens today to a patient with simple indigestion and heart burn. If he goes to an internist or family physician, the typical history of indigestion and heart burn, most often relieved by antacids, is elicited. Physical examination usually reveals slight tenderness in the epigastrium (the upper abdomen just below the breast bone). The physician will prescribe an acid suppressant, perhaps a special diet and see the patient in 2-4 weeks. At that time, the typical patient will tell the doctor he's entirely asymptomatic. The only question remaining is the length of time the patient should remain on the medication and when it's stopped, whether there is a recurrence. The average patient remains on the medication for 6-8 weeks.

Now if this same patient opts to go to a gastroenterologist, he will initially have a complete physical examination with laboratory work that will quadruple the initial cost. He will then be advised that endoscopy is necessary. This entails the introduction of a flexible scope down the esophagus into the stomach and duodenum. The usual finding will be some degree of inflammation. The scoping itself can cost anywhere from $200.00 to $350.00 and subjects the patient to a procedure that might cause an esophageal tear, which is a disaster. The patient is told he has areas of inflammation in his stomach and duodenum. Didn't the patient know that already? Inflammation causes heartburn, indigestion, and spasm. The patient is then placed on an acid suppressant and the scoping is repeated in 6 weeks. He is then told the inflammation is all gone. But the patient knows that already because he has been asymptomatic within 2-3 days after the introduction of the acid suppressant.

The cost: 6 weeks of care by the internist or family physician is approximately $150.00, versus 6 weeks of therapy by the gastroenterologist, approximately $800.00-$900.00.

The simple rule that many gastroenterologists ignore is: Don't scope unless the patient doesn't improve. Of course, if you don't scope you are not handsomely rewarded.

A similar example could be given for every field of medicine. The solution to the problem is simple: there has to be a generalist in charge of the patient (not the government or an insurance company).

Chapter Seventeen

A Mess in the Garage

*I*t seemed the phone was ringing constantly. Heaven must be a place without buzzers or bells, I thought.

"Hello, Doctor?"

"Yes, this is the Doctor," I said wearily, every muscle in my body sagging with fatigue.

I had been going at a maniacal pace since five in the morning when I had seen that bleeding ulcer in the emergency room of the hospital.

"I'm so glad I caught you, Doctor."

The youthful vitality of the voice made my shoulders droop even more.

"Is there something wrong?" I said, sitting at my desk and pushing back the mountain of forms the nurse had deposited there.

"You sound tired, Doctor."

"I am exhausted," I said. "I don't have the strength to lift a pencil. Did you call to tell me my voice sounds tired?"

"Oh no, Doctor. I'm sorry if I'm interrupting you. This is Ruth Henderson."

"Ruthie, I thought your voice sounded familiar. I hope nothing's wrong. Are you having a problem?"

"I'm fine, Doctor. I'm not calling about myself. It's George. Well, it's...sort of a delicate matter. I really don't know how to begin. Perhaps I should come down to the office?"

"Is George sick, Ruthie?"

"That's the problem, Doctor, I really and honestly don't know. But I'm desperate. I need your advice badly. You know, it's one of those times that I just can't think straight. I suppose if I was religious, I'd go see a priest or minister or light a candle, but I don't think anything like that would help much when I need action right now. I think I'm just going to panic and tear my hair out and eat ten chocolate bars."

"Now Ruthie, take hold of yourself. You're not going to panic or tear your hair out or any other foolish thing. After all, I've known you since I delivered you into this beautiful agony called 'Our World' and you haven't panicked yet, have you?"

"No, I haven't, Doctor, thanks to you. But this time it's different. I just have to come down to talk to you. If I don't, I think I'll get drunk or just go out of my bloody mind. Have you ever had one of those days?"

"I have one every day, Ruthie."

"Well, I guess you do, Doctor. But I'm not used to that kind of stress. I'm about ready to jump off the nearest bridge."

I looked at my watch, temporarily forgetting my fatigue.

"It's 4:30 now, Ruthie. Come in at 5:30. We'll talk about George and anything else that's bothering you. Remember now, 5:30."

"I love you, Doctor. You're the greatest. I'll be there 5:30 sharp. I don't think I could live without you."

"5:30 sharp, Ruthie."

I hung up the phone, feeling old right down to the balls of my feet. I remembered delivering Ruthie twenty-two years ago and George four years before that, just as if those events had occurred a few weeks ago. I hated to think of them as anything but permanent children.

I had one hour before Ruthie's appointment and old Mrs. Lena Danton was still out in the waiting room.

"I'm so glad you came today, Lena," I said, kissing her on the cheek. "I would have been very upset if you hadn't stopped by before moving to Maine."

Lena smiled.

"Thirty years, Doctor," she said. "You've been taking care of me for all of thirty years and I certainly couldn't leave town without saying good-by."

"The amazing thing, Lena," I said, as I flipped through her thick chart, "is that nothing I ever prescribed for you over all those years ever worked on you."

"That *is* amazing, isn't it, Doctor?" Lena said, looking wide-eyed. "But you took such good care of me during all those miserable times I had and you never got upset once when I'd call you up to tell you the medicine you prescribed made me worse. I'm just like my mother was, allergic to everything, bless her soul. She couldn't tolerate any kind of medicine, either. The thing I'll always remember about you, Doctor, as long as I live, is that you always took the time to listen to me even when I brought in those long lists of complaints that I had written out. You'd go over every one of them with me, one by one, even when you had a waiting room full of patients. I do hope I find another doctor like you in Greenville."

"I'm sure you will, Lena, and as soon as you do I'll send your medical records to him."

She leaned over for another peck on the cheek. I hugged her. There were tears in her eyes.

"Don't forget to write, Lena," I said as she left awkwardly, trying to conceal her crying.

She was an elegant lady.

I checked a few urine specimens deposited by patients during the afternoon, signed several insurance forms, and then called in about a dozen prescriptions to local pharmacies.

The hour melted away rapidly and finally Ruthie was there sitting opposite me in her tiny miniskirt with her legs crossed, showing an expanse of thigh practically up to her buttocks. She looked upset and couldn't sit still.

"This time I know it's a really serious problem, Doctor," she said, brushing the hair from her face. "I'm not calling wolf like the time George couldn't get an erection and I thought the world was coming to an end. I think George has really flipped his wig."

She uncrossed her legs, lit a cigarette, squinted through the smoke, put out the cigarette after she spied the no smoking sign, recrossed her legs, and finally balanced herself on her left buttock.

"Tell me about it, Ruthie, and take your time. Tell me everything."

She was like a daughter to me.

"Well, you know George, Doctor. He's been a rebel all his life, just a natural-born protester, I suppose you'd call him. It must be in his genes."

"Yes, that's George, Ruthie, just as we both know him. When he was born I practically had to pry him out of his mother's womb and yank him out by his feet. He had to come into this world rear-end first. I remember his clavicle broke in the process. And when he was baptized, he urinated in the holy water, an unmistakable sign of a true protester."

"That was his first protest but not his last, Doctor, as you well know. I wouldn't have been surprised if he had been born carrying a placard denouncing the world and the Establishment. But this time I think he's gone too far. I didn't mind when he backed McCarthy for president and worked for him in New Hampshire. Even when he switched to Bobby Kennedy, that was OK with me. Then we managed to live through the Democratic convention riots in Chicago. Now, of course, it's the contamination of the environment and a million other things. But his present protest, I think, is just too much for me to take. This time he has gone too far. You know it isn't easy being married to a natural-born protester."

"I know, Ruthie, I know. Exactly what has he done?"

"I don't even know how to start...it's sort of embarrassing."

"Remember Ruthie, I have heard just about everything any doctor could ever hear. Don't be embarrassed. Tell me in simple words. What has George done this time?"

"For the past three nights, Doctor, George has come home and asked me for the editorial page of *The New York Times.*"

"What's so odd about that, Ruthie? George has read *The Times* for years."

"Yes, I know, I know. Nothing's odd about that. But then he goes to the bathroom—but not in the bathroom."

"How's that again?"

"He goes to the bathroom, but not in the bathroom."

"I thought you said that, Ruthie."

"That's exactly what he does. He takes the editorial page of *The Times* and goes out into the garage and goes to the bathroom."

"You mean he goes out into the garage and squats and...and..."

"Yes, he does. Now don't you think he's carrying his protests a little too far for his own good?"

"You mean you think he's protesting the editorial policy of *The Times*, Ruthie?"

"What else, Doctor? You know how violent he gets about some of those editorials. I wouldn't mind it so much if he asked for the Sears and Roebuck catalog once in a while, or the funnies. But no, it's always the editorial page of *The Times*. Now that certainly isn't normal behavior, is it, Doctor?"

"In this day and age, Ruthie, I wouldn't try to define normal behavior. But I do have to admit it appears to be somewhat unusual behavior, to say the least. Even for George."

"And if that isn't enough, Doctor, George then proceeds to take a stick and mess around with his protest. God, if he wants to make mud pies, I'll get him some silly putty. I really can't take much more of this."

"George has always been an unusual character, Ruthie. You knew that when you married him. I wouldn't be at all surprised to hear that you helped him out on a few of his wild adventures. Isn't that true, Ruthie?"

"Yes, I did, Doctor, and I'm ashamed to admit it. But now he has gone too far. You know that I'm broad-minded and I can tolerate a lot of screwball activities, but what if he decides to do something like this in public?"

"I don't think that George would ever carry his protests that far, Ruthie. There may be some simple explanation for this unusual behavior that you and I are missing. Did you confront him about this matter?"

"Heck, no! I thought I'd better speak to you first. He's got me so mixed up the other day I put gin in my douche bag instead of white vinegar. I nearly went into orbit. We make a great pair, George out in the garage messing around with his protest and me with gin in my douche bag."

"Well, I'm glad you came down to speak to me about this, Ruthie. Has George been ill lately?"

"No, he hasn't. He's as strong as a bull."

"Has he had any unusual illnesses in his lifetime, Ruthie?"

"You should know the answer to that better than anybody on this earth, Doctor. You delivered him and took care of him when he was sick."

"I mean during the times he's been away from home attending college or going on some of these protest rallies. You can meet a lot of odd people with a variety of medical conditions when you leave the security of your own home town."

"No. As far as I know, he's had just the usual childhood diseases like measles, mumps, chicken pox, and gonorrhea. You remember his mother didn't believe in vaccination."

"Has he ever protested anything in this manner before, Ruthie?"

"The only time I can think of was in his senior year in college. He and a bunch of his classmates all got C in Physiology, and that night they went over to Professor Compton's house after drinking all the beer they could find in their fraternity house."

She paused and looked out the window.

"Yes," I said. "Go on."

"It's really all so stupid and juvenile," she said. "They emptied their bladders on Professor Compton's front lawn and then howled at the moon like a bunch of banshees. Grass never grows there ever since they started this ritual. Now he and his classmates make a pilgrimage to that very spot every five years as part of their reunion activities."

"Well, in college we can excuse a lot of things, Ruthie, even that. But George is older now and is rapidly becoming a member of the Establishment."

"This present activity is something I really can't understand, Doctor. I've gone over everything in our past to see if I could find some clue to help me understand this. But there's nothing, nothing at all, to help me explain his present activities."

"Does he appear stressed out?"

"He has been up-tight lately, nervous as a cat, practically hyper-thyroid, and blowing his cool constantly. And for no reason. We're making plenty of money and all our bills are paid. He hasn't done anything stupid for at least six months. Then wham, bam, right out of the blue. Damn, damn *The New York Times*."

"Ruthie, now listen to me. We have to get George down here on some pretext. I have to talk to him before something really serious happens."

"But he's healthy and strong as a bull, Doctor. I can't think of anything that would make him come down here to talk to you."

"We must think of something to get him down here, Ruthie. Otherwise, there is no way on this earth to help him. We certainly can't abduct him by force or hospitalize him against his will. Perhaps you can drop something on his big toe or step on it accidentally."

"I'll think of something, Doctor, don't worry. I'll get him down here if it's the last thing I do."

She stood up, hoisting her panty hose, the crotch having slipped too low. With a final adjustment of her miniskirt to just below her buttocks, she stood in front of me ready to go, her pretty face drawn with worry.

"Thank you, Doctor. Now that I've told you everything, I feel better. If you can't help my poor George, then nobody can. I'll get him down here even if I have to bite him."

"You get him down here, Ruthie, and I'll take care of the rest. Don't worry."

She bounced out of the room, half-smiling, half-worried, not knowing whether to cry or laugh.

The next night, I had just sat down to start my supper when the phone rang. No matter what time I ate supper it was always the same.

"Hello," I said wearily, swallowing some potato salad at the same time.

"That you, Doctor?"

"Yes. Is that you, George?"

"Yes. This is George Henderson. I'm surprised that you recognized my voice. I haven't seen you for a few years."

"I remember all the babies I've delivered, George. They're like my own children."

There was a long pause and I could hear George breathing.

"How are you, Doctor?"

"Is that why you called, George, to inquire about my health?"

"No, Doctor. I hate to bother you during supper time, but I need your help badly."

"Good, George, good...well, I mean...you're not sick, are you, George?"

"No, I'm not really sick, but I'll tell you, I'm scared to death."

"About what, George?"

"I really can't tell you over the phone, Doctor. It's sort of a delicate problem. Do you think I could come down to the office? I know you don't have office hours tonight but I'm desperate."

"Everybody's desperate these days, George," I said. "It's part of the times, a universal panic syndrome. It's the way we live."

"I don't mean that kind of being desperate. I mean personally desperate."

"You mean you have a personal problem, George?"

"Yes, personal and anatomical, and maybe even physiological."

"All right, George. I'll meet you at my office in one hour. And George..."

"Yes, Doctor?"

"Take it real easy, George. I'm sure we'll be able to solve your problem."

"I hope so, Doctor. You're talking to a man standing on the lip of a volcano."

"One hour, George."

I finished supper, called in some prescriptions, and one hour later met a frightened George Henderson at my office. He sat opposite me silently, looking down at the floor and fiddling with the cap he held in his hands.

"Well, George," I finally said after a few minutes, "we came here to talk. Tell me what's bothering you."

"I don't know how to begin, Doctor. I'm scared silly."

"Just start at the beginning, George, and tell me the whole thing. You'll feel better once you get it off your chest."

"To tell you the truth, Doctor, the whole thing started at a protest march."

"What were you protesting about this specific time, George?"

"The editorial policy of *The New York Times*."

"Now we're getting somewhere, George."

"Do you realize, Doctor, that if *The Times* hadn't suppressed the leak about the Bay of Pigs affair and had gone ahead like a responsible newspaper printing the story, well, the Bay of Pigs fiasco simply wouldn't have taken place?"

"Yes, I suppose so, George. I really haven't followed the news that closely. That's why I think protesters like you are so vital to our democratic system because you people get involved in things I don't have time to even think about. But tell me, exactly how did this affect you personally?"

"That's how I met Claudia, Doctor."

"Claudia! Who's Claudia, George, and what has she got to do with your problem?"

"That's what I'm getting to. Claudia is a natural-born protester just like me. We are alike as any two condoms in a package of three. In fact, she happened to be born with a fractured clavicle like I was. So there we were, two cognate souls marching together for the common good of society. The next thing I knew, my hand was up her miniskirt."

"While you were marching, George? My God."

"No, of course not, Doctor. It was later. That's when I found out she never wore any underclothes of any kind. No panties, no bra. The first completely free woman I ever met. I felt like Shelley when they were preaching free love in England in 1810. It was an alliance made in heaven."

"Horse shit, George."

"What was that again, Doctor? I didn't quite hear you."

"Horse shit, George. That's pure horse shit."

George looked down at his shoes.

"Well, anyway," George said, "it all began as a swimming date, skinny dipping. I just lost my head completely and forgot all about Ruthie and everything else in the world. I didn't even give a damn about the editorial policy of *The Times*. That's how far gone I was. Getting Claudia in the sack became the most important goal in my life."

"This story is getting a familiar ring to it, George."

"That's it exactly, Doctor. The rings. We were in the water when she remembered she had left her rings on. They were sort of loose, both her engagement ring and her wedding ring because she had been dieting. She was afraid she was going to lose them, so she took them off and gave them to me. Like a stupid ass, I put them in my mouth and began to swim to shore. A wave caught me just right and I swallowed the damn things."

"You swallowed both the rings, George?"

"Yes, and now I'm scared to death."

"Don't worry, George. You'll pass them without any trouble."

"You're sure, Doctor? It's three days and I haven't passed them yet. You're sure I won't have to be scoped?"

"I'm sure, George. Have you checked to make sure you haven't passed them already?"

"Yes, I have. In a complete panic. Every night for the past three nights, I go out into the garage, spread some paper on the floor, do my duty, and then poke around with a stick."

"Oh, so that's what you've been doing...I mean...so that's what modern technology has come down to."

"Can you think of a better way, Doctor, considering the circumstances?"

"No, I can't, George. And you haven't found them yet?"

"No."

"Maybe you missed them, George. Three days is a long time."

"A lot longer than seventy-two hours, Doctor. I'll tell you that. What have you got planned for me?"

"First, we'll get an x-ray of your abdomen, George. And if the rings are still there, I'll give you a cathartic to end all cathartics. And they will pass, I promise you. Don't worry another moment. Your problem is as good as solved."

"Claudia is after me constantly about the rings. Her husband hasn't noticed that they're missing yet. If I get out of this with my skin in one piece, it'll be a miracle."

"These miracles are brought about in this office every day, George. Your problem is solved, I tell you."

I scheduled an abdominal x-ray for George the next day. I put the films up on the view box.

"There they are, George, in all their glory," I said. "They're still in your stomach."

"Jesus Christ," George said, shaking his head. "If this keeps up any longer, I'm sure Ruth will get suspicious about my activities in the garage."

"Stop worrying, George. Take this prescription and you'll probably pass them tomorrow. In the meantime, keep doing your duty in the garage when Ruthie isn't home. By the way, what newspaper do you get at home?"

"*The New York Times*, Doctor. Why do you want to know that?"

"Do you use any particular page when you do your job in the

garage?"

"I read the editorial page last, so that's the one I usually use."

"Use a different part of the paper, George. Maybe your luck will change."

"I'll do anything to get those rings, Doctor. If Claudia's husband ever notices the rings are missing, he'll beat the hell out of me. He's got a violent temper."

"You should pass them within the next twenty-four hours, George. Keep doing your garage work. Make believe you're working on the car."

"You know, Doctor, I'm surprised."

"Why, George?"

"You must be superstitious if you think changing the page will have an effect on my bowels."

"I'm superstitious when I have to be, George. I'd even resort to voodoo if I thought it would work."

"So would I, Doctor."

The following day, George came into the office again. He looked terrible.

"They didn't pass, Doctor. I didn't sleep all night. Please take another x-ray just to see if they have started their journey yet."

I tried to talk him out of another x-ray but he was nearly hysterical. The x-ray tech completed the procedure and put the films on the view box.

"They have started their journey, George. Finally. Take another dose of that cathartic tonight and we'll be in Diamond City tomorrow."

"I hope so, Doctor. I don't think I can hold out much longer."

"You'll hold out as long as necessary, George. We're almost home."

About an hour later, Ruth Henderson was on the phone.

"I've got good news for you, Ruthie."

"Oh, thank God."

"George is going to be all right. Just a little bowel trouble, that's all. He'll have to be careful about what he puts into his mouth. Cut out all the rich stuff and the junk food."

"I love you, Doctor. You're the greatest."

"Any news from that end, Ruthie?"

"Nothing except George is now using the front page of *The Times*. Do you think that means anything?"

"I think we're making progress, Ruthie. Any day now, George should be all over his troubles."

The next day George was at my office with a big smile. He hugged me.

"I love you like my father, Doctor."

"Keep the faith, George."

"I delivered the rings to the owner. This whole thing shook Claudia up so badly she began to wear underwear. Her husband never noticed the rings were missing. And what's more, I've decided to give up protest marches and rock festivals and skinny-dipping for a while."

"Good boy, George. Not one of my babies has gone bad yet, but I'll tell you I was worried about you for awhile."

"I've learned my lesson, Doctor."

"That's what life is all about, George."

About two hours later, Ruth Henderson was on the phone.

"I could kiss you, Doctor." She made the sound of a big wet smooch. "I love you, I love you, I love you. You're the greatest ever. George used the bathroom for the first time in a week. I mean to say he went to the bathroom in the bathroom. You know what I mean."

"I know what you mean, Ruthie. I knew George would come through this crisis intact."

"And you know what, Doctor?"

"No, what, Ruthie?"

"George canceled his subscription to *The Times*. I can't help but believe that may have been the cause of his whole problem. Damn that newspaper. Damn, damn *The New York Times*."

About three months later, I unfolded the local newspaper to see a picture of George and Ruth Henderson on the front page with the following caption: "Local residents take part in protest march at nuclear power plant."

Because Ruthie was with George on this protest, I knew that I wouldn't have to worry about another mess in the garage.

LESSONS TO BE LEARNED

It is obvious that the doctor and the young couple enjoyed a unique relationship. He treated them like his own special children and they treated him like an honored uncle for whom they had great respect and even more than that because they were willing to discuss the most intimate details of their lives. It is rare for a specialist to develop this type of relationship with his patients because it takes years of constant and renewed bonding. Unfortunately, this type of close relationship can be a trap because when disaster strikes patients like this, it may result in an emotional crisis which if repeated frequently enough, may render the physician hopelessly mired in chronic depression.

As for Lena Danton, she was a grand lady. All she needed in a doctor was a good listener. She actually hated to take medicine of any kind. Fortunately, she was basically a strong, healthy woman and required very little attention. She came willingly into the office to alert the physician that she was under attack by the various minor diseases she suffered. Once he was alerted and she felt she was under his care, she then allowed all her medical problems to run their natural courses, never suffering any significant complications. Her mother lived to be 102 years old and I suspected that Lena would easily reach that venerable age, too.

She was smart enough to pick a physician who didn't allow his ego to interfere with good judgment when told his prescriptions made her worse, or when she preferred to let her own body's defenses solve her problems.

Chapter Eighteen

An Incidental Perforation

Mrs. Florence Higgenbotham sat in the chair next to the desk and looked at me suspiciously, her arms folded across her ample bosom. She was a big woman, six feet tall and two hundred fifty pounds. Her husband sat to her right. He was a small man, five feet four and one hundred ten.

"What can I do for you folks?" I said, not sure who the patient was.

"Mrs. Higgenbotham would like a blood sugar," Mr. Higgenbotham said, looking at his wife for her approval.

Mrs. Higgenbotham nodded her head slightly.

"Are you a diabetic, Mrs. Higgenbotham?" I said.

"No, she isn't," Mr. Higgenbotham said. "At least not yet, anyway. Her sister is, however."

"Do you have any symptoms at the present time, Mrs. Higgenbotham?" I said.

"Mrs. Higgenbotham has developed excessive thirst over the past three months," Mr. Higgenbotham said. "She also urinates frequently and has started to lose weight."

"As you probably already know, those are the classic symptoms of diabetes mellitus," I said. "I'll have the nurse get you ready for a brief examination and I'll take a more detailed history. Then, I'll check your urine and do a blood sugar test, Mrs. Higgenbotham."

"No, you don't understand, Doctor," Mr. Higgenbotham said. "All Mrs. Higgenbotham wants is a simple blood sugar. She is fearful and suspicious of all doctors. Basically, I guess I have to say it, she just doesn't like doctors."

Again, Mrs. Higgenbotham nodded her head slightly. I hesitated a moment.

"All right," I said. "This is unusual, but if that's all Mrs. Higgenbotham wants, that's all she's going to get. I'll send the nurse in to draw your blood, Mrs. Higgenbotham. I notice your husband is doing all the talking, but I assume you can speak. Is that correct?"

"Oh, yes, good Lord, she can speak up a storm," Mr. Higgenbotham said. "When she gets going, nothing can stop her tongue, just like any woman."

Mrs. Higgenbotham's eyes shifted sternly to her husband. I knew he would be in for it when they got home.

"What I mean to say, Doctor, is that Mrs. Higgenbotham does the thinking in our house and I do the talking. Isn't that right, dear?"

Again that barely perceptible nod came from Mrs. Higgenbotham.

"Well, I would like to hear you say something, Mrs. Higgenbotham," I said. "Otherwise, I would have to describe you in my office records as being mute."

"Mute!" Mr. Higgenbotham said abruptly, unable to repress a laugh. "That's a good one, Doctor. You should hear this woman talk at home. Why, sometimes I think she'll never stop. Oh, she can talk all..."

Mrs. Higgenbotham gave her husband a look that would have turned an ordinary mortal into stone and he stopped suddenly.

"Yes, I can speak, Doctor, but only when it's necessary. I'm a woman of very few words."

At that, Mr. Higgenbotham snorted, coughed, wheezed, and finally pulled out his handkerchief and hid his face.

"Usually, I have Mr. Pipsqueak here, who apparently is convulsing, speak for me," Mrs. Higgenbotham continued. "And frequently, he ends up by saying too much."

She sat in her chair, eyebrows furrowed, looking sternly at her husband. He turned away from her.

The nurse came in and drew the blood. The blood sugar was was 250 mgm.

"Do you want me to give Mrs. Higgenbotham the results," the nurse said, as she handed me the report, "or are you going to talk with her yourself, Doctor?"

"I think I'd better go in and talk to them myself, even though they already told me she doesn't want to be examined."

I went in and gave them the results of the blood sugar.

"Do you have any questions, Mrs. Higgenbotham?" I said. "I'd be glad to discuss the significance of this blood sugar if you like, and what we can do to bring it down within the normal range. You know, in order to have a proper doctor-patient relationship, it's important to have trust and confidence in your doctor. I'd feel very unhappy if you didn't allow me to discuss your problem with you."

Mr. Higgenbotham looked at Mrs. Higgenbotham for direction but she remained silent.

"It might be a good idea if you gave us some advice, Doctor," Mr. Higgenbotham said finally.

I gave them a brief explanation of diabetes mellitus and the importance of diet and exercise.

"A doctor once said that the best way to achieve a long, healthy life is to develop a mild, chronic illness and then take care of it properly. The type of mild diabetes you have fits that description nicely and with proper care, Mrs. Higgenbotham, I know that you'll do well."

"I don't believe that Mrs. Higgenbotham has diabetes, Doctor," Mr. Higgenbotham said. "She just has a high blood sugar."

"An elevated blood sugar," I continued, "can seriously affect your eyes, your heart, your kidneys, and your circulation. Even your nervous system can be involved. I would be surprised if you haven't been having blurring of your vision, Mrs. Higgenbotham."

It took me over an hour of gentle persuasion to overcome her fear. She finally relented and allowed me to perform a brief examination of her heart, lungs, blood pressure, eyes, and the circulation in her feet.

"Everything appears to be in order, Mrs. Higgenbotham," I said.

"See, just as I thought," Mr. Higgenbotham said. "The exam was really unnecessary since everything's normal."

"How would we have known that, Mr. Higgenbotham," I said, "unless we had done the exam?"

Mrs. Higgenbotham censured her husband with her eyes again.

Over the following months, Mrs. Higgenbotham gradually lost her fear of the office and allowed me to do a complete physical examination; everything except a pelvic and rectal. Her blood sugar came down within normal range merely on diet and exercise. A few months later, she told me she was ready for the first pelvic and rectal examinations she had ever had. Unfortunately, the pap smear was abnormal, revealing a carcinoma of the lining of the uterus, the endometrium.

"I knew we should never have started coming to the doctor," Mr. Higgenbotham said. "He's finding more and more things wrong with you."

I referred her to a gynecologist.

She was admitted three days later and a D and C was scheduled for the following day. This procedure consists of dilating the cervix, which is the narrow neck of the uterus, and then scraping the lining of the uterus clean with a curette. I wrote the initial history and physical examinations in the chart. The lab work was all normal. The fasting blood sugar was 120 mgm%. This is the upper limit of normal. Mrs. Higgenbotham achieved this without any great effort.

"I knew she didn't have diabetes," Mr. Higgenbotham said.

The D and C started out without any problems, but during the procedure, the gynecologist put too much pressure on the curettte and punctured the wall of the uterus, spilling the cancerous endometrium into the abdominal cavity. The operation ended up being an emergency hysterectomy instead of a simple diagnostic D and C.

When I came in to see her the next day, Mrs. Higgenbotham was crying. Mr. Higgenbotham was still home and she had to speak for herself.

"I don't want another operation, Doctor," she said, crying softly.

"What are you talking about, Mrs. Higgenbotham?" I said. "You're not scheduled for more surgery."

"Oh, yes I am," she said. "Dr. Skinner was just in and he told me he found my gall bladder was full of stones and another surgeon has scheduled gall bladder surgery in three days. I really don't think I can stand another operation this soon, do you?"

Mrs. Higgenbotham had never had a gall bladder attack and Dr. Skinner hadn't bothered to discuss further surgery with me. This created an awkward situation.

"You aren't going to have another operation, Mrs. Higgenbotham, I promise you. You've never had a gall bladder attack and your chances of having one are just about zero. I'll speak to the surgeon and get everything straightened out. In a few days you'll be going home to Mr. Pipsqueak, excuse me, I mean your husband and you'll feel much better. Now please stop crying and concentrate on getting better."

A slight smile played briefly across her face amid her tears when I called her husband Mr. Pipsqueak.

"Thank you, Doctor. I knew I could count on you. And to think at one time I didn't trust doctors. Of course, I have to admit I still don't, but that doesn't include you."

Mrs. Higgenbotham recovered nicely from her surgery but six months later, she had a generalized seizure. A CT scan revealed the cancer in her uterus had metastasized to her brain. She died a month later.

We had caught the original cancer at an early stage. However, the perforation of the uterus during the D and C had disseminated the tumor throughout her abdominal cavity and it finally metastasized to her brain. Neither the gynecologist nor the general surgeon was pleased with the fact that I canceled the gall bladder surgery. I wasn't happy with what they had planned to do, either.

I often wondered how long Mrs. Higgenbotham would have lived if she had allowed her fears and suspicions to control her destiny and had never gone to see a doctor. As for her husband, Mr. Pipsqueak, I never saw him again.

LESSONS TO BE LEARNED

Many patients will try to limit a physician's participation in his or her care to such an extent that it would be ludicrous to accept the responsibility without performing, at least, the minimum examination. Even though the patient may not admit it, fear is usually behind this type of problem. If the physician is extremely busy, he could easily dismiss the patient abruptly, stating that he is not willing to accept a patient for treatment on such restricted terms.

But if he does this, has the physician helped the patient in any way? And then if the patient is dismissed in this manner, walks outside and drops dead, that surely would result in some fine courtroom discussion. Part of a physician's obligation is to help the individual overcome his fear. It's true that the doctor might have to spend more time with the patient. Not everybody can be fortunate enough to have the patient anesthetized before he starts his work. Sometimes a primary physician has to tread a path around obstacles deliberately set by patients to impede the progress of the physician instead of helping him.

It takes much longer to elicit an adequate history when the husband and wife are in the office together. The sooner the physician realizes that and allows extra time, the less anxious he'll be about getting on with other work waiting and piling up.

A common problem that a physician faces in practice occurs when a patient is referred to a surgeon, and the surgeon then refers the patient to another physician without first discussing the problem with the original doctor. An awkward situation can easily develop as it did in this case. It was unethical for the gynecologist to refer this patient for further surgery without calling me. The sad part is that many surgeons become angry when an internist or family physician interferes with their carefully laid plans.

As for the perforation, that was inexcusable, and was the main reason for the early metastases and subsequent death of this patient.

Chapter Nineteen

Jabber O'Houlihan

Jabber O'Houlihan didn't earn his nickname by being silent. He was a little man and a big talker. Anybody within earshot could hear his mouth going constantly. And if nobody happened to be there, he would talk to himself. He would ad lib both sides of the conversation, often singing snatches of melodies, limericks, and poetry. There was a constant flow of words from his mouth, cast upon the air currents to be swept away in all directions. And whenever he happened upon a choice phrase, he would cock his head to one side and narrow his eyes and say, "Now, did you hear that fine phrase, Mr. Sean O'Casey? As fine a phrase as you will ever hear on this earth."

After each "fine phrase," Jabber would have a swallow of beer. As he continued to drink, the flow of words increased, and by the end of the evening, Sean O'Casey would have a whole new lexicon of phrases, cast out on a beery breath only to be forgotten. Among the drinkers in town, Jabber was recognized as the undisputed champion of the beer lovers, the king, a little man with a big thirst.

He worked as a tool-and-die maker at the old Marlin-Rockwell plant on Woodford Avenue from seven to four every day. In spite of his drinking habits, he never missed a day's work and was proud of that fact. But at four on the dot, his tongue stuck so fiercely to his hard palate he could only speak in a hoarse whisper, he would scurry across the street to O'Neil's Bar and Grill. He'd order his first Bud, and like a miracle, his tongue would become unglued from his hard palate, and the words would begin their majestic march from his mouth.

He ran book on all the sporting events and managed to earn enough to pay for his beer and all the beer for his friends. For that reason, the betting was fast and furious at times. Even if a customer was a heavy loser, he knew he could recoup his losses in beer.

Jabber usually started home by seven o'clock in the evening. Occasionally, when the crowd of men was especially big and the betting was heavy, he wouldn't get away until eight or nine. By then, he was fully tanked and wouldn't be able to walk a straight line. Not that he had any desire to. Because of his heavy drinking, he was inclined to fall frequently. On some occasions, he would appear completely battered and his friends would accuse him of losing another round to his wife.

"The little lady loves me and would never stoop low enough to strike a man who is temporarily indisposed," Jabber would counter.

One day he walked all the way home with one foot in the gutter and the other on the sidewalk, cursing the men who would dare to lay such an uneven sidewalk in our lovely, little town.

"Another fine example of the graft that exists in the construction industry," he muttered into the wind, burping and passing gas.

When he appeared especially battered, the cops would pick him up and take him to my office. I would admit him to the hospital to prevent him from being arrested and to allow him to dry out. He went through the detox program more than any other individual in town.

"And I don't drink one drop less because of it," he would say as he swallowed more beer. "And that's a record any man could be proud of."

"I suppose, Doctor, my honorable friend," he said during one of those drying-out periods, "that it would be easy to come to the conclusion that the Irish have a reputation for heavy drinking."

"Why, Jabber," I said, feigning astonishment, "whatever made you come to that conclusion?"

"Let me tell you, Doctor, how the poor Irish managed to develop such an outrageous and preposterous reputation, one that is so far from the truth that it's utterly unbelievable."

"Please, Jabber," I said, "please tell me. I've been simply dying to hear the truth regarding that bit of Irish folklore for years."

"Well, sir," Jabber said, "it was St. Patrick's Day a number of years ago that I finally decided to destroy completely that foolish myth of Irish drinking and restore their rightful reputation of temperate, God-fearing citizens totally dedicated to complete abstinence from alcoholic beverages of any kind."

Jabber's body shuddered as he mentioned the word abstinence.

"Are you sure you're talking about the Irish, Jabber," I said.

"As I live and breathe, so help me God, Doctor," Jabber said. "So on this St. Patrick's Day in question, I deputized a team from O'Neil's Bar and Grill and sent them out to all the Irish pubs within a radius of ten miles from the very spot where we're standing. Every man who entered the pub was obliged to sign his name and address on a special register. Sure enough, as I expected, every name was Irish. There were Scanlons, O'Ryans, Cohans, O'Tooles, Tobins, Cavanaughs, McDougals, Calahans, O'Shaughnessys, Kilpatricks, and so forth."

"You've just proved the point you started out to disprove, Jabber," I said.

"Hold on there, my honorable Doctor," Jabber said. "I haven't finished my soliloquy. As each of these so-called Irishmen departed from the pubs, I had one of my deputies follow him at a discreet distance. And what do you think I found out?"

"I have no idea, Jabber," I said, "but I know it must have been earth-shattering."

"Earth-shattering doesn't even come close to matching the state of stupefaction that I fell into," Jabber said. "Mr. O'Ryan drove up to a house with the name Koslowski on the mailbox; Mr. O'Toole drove up to a house with the name Malichewski on the mailbox; Mr. Cavanaugh ended up in Madowski's house and so on and so on. Everyone of these men who had drunk to excess on St. Patrick's Day turned out to be Polish. This information shatters all the myths about the Irish being the biggest drinkers on this planet. The Polish now have that title and God bless them for being so devoted to that heavenly brew."

"Now I know why they call you Jabber," I said.

Jabber O'Houlihan finally got into serious trouble one day as he was driving past my office. He later said that some kind of optical illusion developed after he left O'Neil's Bar and Grill and the road suddenly narrowed. It may have been the light reflected from the stained-glass windows of the Episcopal Church across the street. He sideswiped five cars that were parked in front of my office.

He stopped his car about thirty feet beyond the last car and sat there as if in a trance. The police found him looking straight ahead, speechless for the first time in his life.

"If you don't hospitalize him, Doctor," the policeman said, "I'll have to arrest him."

I examined Jabber. He was so drunk he could barely move. I admitted him to the hospital and left orders for him to be watched carefully. I didn't get to the hospital until seven o'clock that evening to recheck Jabber. He was lying in bed with his eyes closed, mumbling to himself.

"You're in real trouble this time, Jabber," I said.

"I've got a hole in my sock, Mr. Sean O'Casey," Jabber said, opening his eyes wide, as if he were frightened.

"You don't have your socks on, Jabber," I said.

"Where am I?" Jabber said. "Did my sister Mary call you?"

"You're in the hospital, Jabber," I said. "Don't you remember hitting those cars? Your sister Mary died five years ago from tuberculosis."

"Mary's dead?" Jabber said surprised. "Why didn't they tell me? My dear sweet sister."

Jabber started to cry. He was obviously under the influence of alcohol and I knew I wouldn't be able to talk to him intelligently until the following day.

The next morning, he seemed much better as we started to talk.

"I guess I really did a job on those cars in front of your office, Doctor," he said.

"You certainly did," I said.

"Did my sister call you?"

"Your sister Mary died five years ago," I said.

Jabber looked at me momentarily confused.

"Why are we talking about Mary, Doctor? You know she died five years ago."

I ordered x-rays of Jabber's skull. CT scans were not available at that time. I removed a sample of his spinal fluid for examination. The x-rays were normal and the spinal fluid had three white cells where there should have been none. I called Dr. Whitford at the city hospital and transferred Jabber to the neurosurgical service there. Dr. Whitford called me back two hours later.

"Your patient is entirely asymptomatic and well-oriented," he said. "He looks great. His neurological exam is entirely normal and his verbal responses are proper. His skull x-rays are negative, as you already know. Would you like me to send him back to you or discharge him?"

Dr. Whitford was one of the best neurosurgeons in the state. I had sent him many cases before. I had great respect for his opinion. I also knew that he would listen to me because I had taken care of this patient for many years.

"Neither, Dr. Whitford," I said. "This man is a chronic alcoholic and has fallen on his head many times in the past. I suspect he has a bilateral subdural hematoma. I believe that's the cause of his abnormal responses, and not his alcoholism."

"If you feel strongly enough about your suspicions, I'll go ahead and do a diagnostic burr hole," Dr. Whitford said.

"I would feel greatly relieved if you went ahead with the surgery, Dr. Whitford," I said. "I'm positive you'll find bilateral subdural hematomas."

Dr. Whitford scheduled the surgery for the next day.

He found bilateral subdural hematomas, just as I suspected. In the middle of the large clot there was a pure culture of Salmonella, which surprised us both.

Jabber made an uneventful recovery. On discharge, the only medication he had to take was Dilantin to prevent convulsive seizures.

He went back to his old habits, drinking every night. After his tenth beer in two hours, he would proclaim himself to be Ignace Jan Paderewski, the famous Polish pianist and statesman.

About two years after his surgery, while walking home from O'Neil's Bar and Grill, he was struck and killed by a drunken driver.

All his cronies from the bar gathered together at his funeral to bid him farewell. After the funeral they hastily retreated to O'Neil's where they proceeded to become very philosophical and melancholy at the thought of losing their friend. That night at the Bar and Grill, a new king was crowned. This time he was Polish. And that undoubtedly made Jabber nod his head in a silent blessing as he gave a sly, knowing wink from his post in the immutable universe.

LESSONS TO BE LEARNED

Alcoholics have an intense desire to be liked. That probably is the main reason they are generally such likable people. I once told one of my alcoholic patients that I had never met an alcoholic that I didn't find congenial. He repeated that statement at his first AA meeting and became an instant success. He never knew he could convince anybody of anything, having restricted his previous talks to his wife. After the reception he received at the AA meeting, he developed a confidence he never had before and spoke at AA meetings throughout the state.

Jabber O'Houlihan didn't think of himself as an alcoholic. Most alcoholics who never miss work feel that single trait is the dividing line separating drunks from "normal people." If Jabber had gone to an AA meeting, he would have been an instant success, too. He also would have invited everybody there to join him at O'Neil's Bar and Grill.

A physician must remember that alcoholics fall frequently. Head injuries in these people are not unusual, even though it's a common belief that an inebriated individual is so relaxed in a fall that he seldom gets hurt.

In this particular case, my hunch that we were dealing with a subdural hematoma was based on the few odd answers that Jabber gave me when I took the initial history. After you've been in practice a number of years, you'll learn to play your hunches because they are based on almost imperceptible evidence that you absorb intuitively. What was surprising was the pure culture of Salmonella in the middle of the clot. Jabber's body had not responded in any way to this abscess because the clot was like a protective envelope preventing the bacteria from attacking the brain.

PATIENT BEWARE—

It's so easy to blame alcohol for every odd symptom or sign observed in drunks. A doctor must be constantly on guard not to fall into this type of trap.

Chapter Twenty

The Hunter

*T*he old man came out on the porch, steadying himself with his cane. It was dark and he barely saw the old dog lying there, pulling himself up slowly with a squeaky yawn.

"Come on, Old Dog," he said. "If we obeyed everything the doctor told us, we'd never get out of this miserable house."

He moved carefully down the steps, his cane tapping. Lord, he thought, it was long in coming. All these months with Charlie nervous as a treed bobcat, building up his courage so slowly that the old man could hardly stand it; and Ella with her fat angry face egging Charlie on.

He remembered the doctor telling him: "Now don't get into any arguments with your daughter-in-law, Ella. Your heart can't take it."

But the doctor was really too busy to spend much time with an old man. And talking certainly wouldn't cure him.

How many times had the old man heard Ella whisper fiercely to Charlie: "When are you going to make him get rid of that dirty old mutt? What's the matter with you? It's only a dog." And Charlie, his face like hard clay, his lips pressed almost bloodless, would just sit there saying nothing.

Then tonight it happened. He had seen it coming in Charlie's eyes. He saw the muscle jumping in his neck.

The old man walked carefully down the street, bent and tired, feeling the cold spread through his body. Already his feet were like two chunks of ice. He heard the dog breathing noisily by his side, wheezing as he expelled the air from his lungs. By the time he reached the corner, the cane tapping out a regular rhythm, he felt the pain in his legs and he stopped to rest.

"Arteriosclerosis, hardening of the arteries," the doctor had said. "They're all plugged up."

Sure, the old man thought, by the time you're seventy-five, if it isn't plugged up, it's shriveled up, and what shouldn't be stiff, is, and what should be stiff, isn't. That's the trick mother nature plays on you.

He kept seeing Charlie's face harsh in the glaring light from the single naked bulb hanging from the kitchen ceiling.

"Me and Ella's been talking, Old Timer, about the dog," Charlie had said. "I know this is your house, but the..."

He never finished the sentence. He didn't have to. He just kept his eyes glued on the piece of wood he was whittling. His voice sounded funny; the words had a difficult time leaving his mouth, as if they were glued inside and had to be pried out with his tongue.

This is it, the old man thought. After all these months of waiting, it's finally here. He stood there feeling tired and old, the knuckles of his right hand white as he leaned hard against the cane.

"I've been trying to think of an easy way to tell you but there ain't any," Charlie said.

No, the old man thought, there never is when you have to squeeze the last drop of blood out of a man.

But now, Charlie's flat rigid monotone kept on like a voice far in the distance and the old man just waited there, weary, hearing the scrape of the knife against the wood. Then the rigid monotone stopped and there was a sudden emptiness and coldness in the room. Even the scraping of the knife had ceased.

It's all over finally, the old man thought. All over and he hadn't even heard the individual words, just the flat sound of Charlie's voice. But he knew it was all over by the frightening silence that followed. The old man shuddered and the monotone started again, relentless and deadly.

"If you don't want to do it yourself, Old Timer, I'll do it for you."

Charlie turned the piece of wood in his hand, examining it carefully, and then blew on it several times. He stood up, brushing the shavings from his pants onto a newspaper that he had spread on the floor. He's brushing me off just like the wood shavings, the old man thought.

He walked slowly out of the kitchen, out of the house past Ella's staring face that was so full of venom and hostility, Charlie's words swirling about him in a fierce mad flight like a bunch of bees.

Then he was out in the cold of the night, resting at the corner, feeling the pain in his legs. He waited a few minutes until the pain subsided and then started walking again. He breathed quickly and hard, as if he couldn't get the air out of his lungs, all the while listening to the dog breathing noisily beside him.

"Emphysema," the doctor had said. "Your lungs are over-expanded and you have a lot of dead space in your chest. Every time you take a breath, it's like putting a bottle of fresh air into a room full of foul air. That's why you're short of breath and you have to breathe quickly."

"Another pleasure of the golden age," he had answered.

By the time he had gotten to the old rusty Thompsonville-Suffield bridge, the pain was stabbing up his legs with severe, wrenching streaks. He rested, leaning against the railing.

You're not so old, Old Dog, he thought. No matter what anybody says. At least not old enough to die yet. By God, I remember when you were just a pup. He laughed quickly at the memory.

"You were a pup, all right," he said, forgetting the pain. "You remember those days down by the old Windsor Locks Canal? Yessir, you really liked the old Canal. In December, the cold would freeze your nose right up. And the banks would be piled high with thick crusts of ice. Those were the days."

The old man closed his eyes and he saw the pup skipping along with his awkward slightly sideways gait. Then the pup stiffened with one paw lifted and the coots would be running furiously, their wings flapping wildly with little circles spreading out where their feet hit the water.

The old man smiled and shook his head. He never could understand why those crazy coots liked to run on the water instead of pushing on it with their wings like a mallard and jumping into the air.

He opened his eyes and laughed again softly to himself.

"By God, you were some pup," he said. "And they said you weren't a dog worth nothing. You remember Pete? How Pete would laugh with his specially trained dogs. He'd near bust a gut laughing. You remember Pete."

The old man was silent then, looking far down the river and listening to the night wind rush softly through the upper structures of the bridge. He shifted his feet and felt the cold in them. The dog leaned against his leg.

"We sure had some fun hunting with Pete, yessir. Down by the Canal and in old man Cavanaugh's corn fields and all those back roads. Those were the days. Pete with his redbones, blueticks, cat hounds, beagles, springers, and pointers. God, what didn't he have? That was Pete. And the way his eyes would bug out when he saw my full bag. Poor Pete."

His face clouded for a moment, his head bobbing slightly. Old Pete died the way a hunter should die, not by inches. There he was, walking up this old dirt road, shotgun ready, hearing his beagle hound pushing in closer, the rabbit bounding into the road and right angle turning. Then the blast and the rabbit flipping high and the excited bark of the hound as he leaped into the road.

The sun was bright that day. He saw Pete turn and smile and then drop dead in the road, the smile still there. That's the way to go, the old man thought. Quick, while you're still active, still hunting, on a perfect day out in the woods.

"You were fast all right, Old Dog. I didn't have a special dog for this or a special dog for that. I just had a special dog."

The dog blinked his wet eyes and cocked his head to one side.

"You're just about the last one I know that I can talk to about the old times, Old Dog. All the others don't seem to understand or don't have the time to listen. Charlie, for instance. Sure, he's a good son and all that but you can see that he really don't care a whittler's damn for hunting. Or fishing, for that matter. I haven't been able to talk to Charlie for years. You know that, Old Dog. As for Ella, she's a woman. The less said about her, the better."

He closed his eyes for a moment, trying to blot out that angry face. He felt the chill of the night air again and shivered.

"I guess we're all getting old, even you, Old Dog."

He looked down at the dog in the dim light.

"You ain't much good now."

The dog cocked his head a little more and looked intently at the old man.

"But by God, I sure remember when you were a pup," the old man said, chuckling to himself. "You were frisky, all right. Just a young pup running around as silly as a dog could be, your whole body twisting and turning just from the sheer joy of being alive. And lord, wetting the bushes every five minutes till I thought you killed them. You even christened old Pete's leg one time and boy, did he growl at you. Silly old dog."

The dog wagged his tail.

"You ain't much good now, though," the old man said. "Useless, that's what you are. Why, you old dog, you can barely move with those arthritic old bones. All you're good for now is for me to scratch your ears. That ain't much good. But you're lucky, you know. At least you still have me to do those things."

The dog licked his hand. Dried crusts curved down from the inner corners of his eyes.

The old man looked up at the clouds moving quickly in the darkening sky. The breeze was getting stiffer.

"I guess you liked rabbit houndin' best, didn't you, Old Dog? You really knew how to track down a jack. What a nose. You remember the frost thick on the ground, and the way you'd jump a bunny, him running crazy for cover and circling slowly back to his form. And all I had to do was wait because I knew there wasn't a rabbit alive that could outsmart you, no matter how much back-tracking, wall-walking, stream-jumping, and fancy stepping he'd try. You'd work slow but sure and there he'd come, circling back to the spot where you flushed him. Like taking candy from a baby, it was."

The old man laughed and patted the dog's head.

"I don't know what's the matter with me tonight. I just can't get old Pete out of my mind. He was a good one, yessir. I still remember the time he was out coon hunting and his favorite bluetick hound caught the scent of a wildcat. What a chase! Old Pete tried everything in the books to call off that dog but the blasted hound was too busy chasing the cat to pay him any mind. The cat would tree and as soon as Pete would come close, he'd be away and gone again with the dog after him and Pete way behind, swearing a bluetick streak. The countryside was full of foul language that night. Well sir, Pete finally ended up in a beaver pond up to his chest in water, and God Almighty, did he swear.''

The old man laughed again. Then he heard the relentless monotone of Charlie's voice and he stood there leaning against the bridge railing, his head bobbing, the pain suddenly heavy in his legs.

I guess Charlie is right, he thought. But the thing that Ella and Charlie forget all the time is that you weren't always old, Old Dog. You were a pup to equal the best. A man shouldn't forget that. Even now, you know how to stand and hold your head.

He looked at the dog and saw the well-formed head with the blunt jaws and the fine long ears. Nothing gives a man more pleasure than having a fine dog, he thought.

How many times had Ella burst out in hot anger at the old man because the dog had dirtied up the house. He couldn't even say a few words in his defense. No sooner would he get out one measly word and whammo, back would come a blast of buckshot that would tear your hide to shreds.

And how many times had he lain in bed listening to Ella's hoarse whisper above the radio. Fierce, angry words that punctured the music like bullet holes, music playing softly, sweetly, so different from her harsh voice, violins so high and muted that he'd remember the wind humming in the electric wires above his head as he walked down miles of railroad track along the river in Enfield. He'd hear the soft drumming of a partridge or the quick flutter of a woodcock rising anxiously out of a tree, sounds that finally drowned out her hellish words. He would sleep then, listening to the dreary whine of the wind in the wires, rising, falling, and his breath would come heavy. Occasionally, he would wake up quickly, knowing that he had stopped breathing. He even mentioned that to the doctor and the doctor explained that kind of breathing was not unusual in elderly people. They even had a special name for it, something that sounded like "chain-smoking" (Cheyne-Stokes respiration). Another great pleasure of old age, he thought, catching yourself not breathing. Who cares, anyway?

Now he stood on the bridge, bent over, tired, trying hard not to think. He started slowly across the bridge, looking at the lights spider-webbed in the upper structures. Just before he reached the other side, he stopped. He leaned over the railing and looked at the black water that hardly seemed to move thirty feet below. He could see the reflections of the bridge lights. They were clear and sharp, but occasionally they would begin to shake as a car passed and he could tell it was water down there and not just empty blackness. Then he listened carefully and he heard the water rush softly around the piers.

"You know, Old Dog," he said. "Straight down the river just about a mile or two, or maybe even closer, the Canal begins. And you know a funny thing about this very spot where we're standing? If you throw a piece of wood into the water from here, it will float right into the Canal sure as we're standing here. Now isn't that something? You really liked the old Canal, didn't you, Old Dog?"

He looked down at the dog and then bent slowly, holding onto the railing, and scratched him behind the ears.

"No, I couldn't do that, Old Dog," he said. "I just couldn't. Not after all we've been through."

He started to walk again and suddenly he realized there was no pain in his legs. He walked faster and took deep breaths of the cool night air. For some reason he felt lighter. He looked at the cane in his right hand and then laughed. He put it under his arm and carried it like a shotgun. He pulled down on his cap and squinted, looking up ahead.

"We'll get a full bag today, don't you worry, Old Dog," he said. "But we'll have to keep moving fast because it looks like we're in for snow."

He stretched out an arm and pointed.

"See that sky. That's snow all right. You can almost smell it in the air."

He kept walking quickly, his legs stretching out, feet striking solidly against the wooden planks of the bridge. The pain was gone out of his thin warped fingers, his knees, his back, his tired and aching muscles. He had no time for pain now. He felt a new power growing quickly, pulsing through him in increasing bursts, fierce with youth, almost jarring his entire body with its strength. He had to get in there fast, get his rabbits, and get out the same way, fast. That blizzard wouldn't wait for anyone.

He thrust his head forward, peering into the blackness, smelling the snow ahead, almost seeing the individual crystals suspended far in the distance, dancing in the cool night air.

"Yessir. Snow. That's snow. A lot of it. Tons of it. White. Blinding. I can smell it. I can almost feel it melt on my skin."

He stretched out his hand and was shocked to feel the coldness. He hadn't expected it to be so close.

It's deceiving, he thought. It had seemed farther away. He strained his eyes peering into the blackness, but it was very dark and he could barely see the outline of his hand that was still stretched out in front of him, feeling the awful cold there.

You really don't have to see the snow to know that it's there. You sense it. Its terrible whiteness surrounds you and presses in on you, making escape impossible. But he was surprised to find it so close. The crystals danced in front of his eyes and yet everything seemed so black.

He came to the end of the bridge and without hesitating, took the narrow path that swung to the left. He felt the stones through the soles of his shoes. He had been a fool to wear those shoes for this kind of weather, but he really hadn't expected the snow. Even the best get fooled at predicting the weather in New England.

The path gradually descended the long sloping bank. He knew every turn, dip, and rise. The river coursed swiftly to his left and he heard the steady rush of the water. He had forgotten the dog momentarily, but now he felt him against his leg and he instinctively bent down and patted him. He finally reached the soft wet dirt by the river. It wasn't long before he saw the dark shadows of the canal locks loom up ahead. The dog breathed noisily behind him but he kept thinking of the snow. He looked up at the sky. That's snow all right.

Suddenly, he felt a heavy crushing weight pressing on his chest. He felt the increasing rushes of pain radiate into his jaw and his left shoulder down to his wrist. He could feel the cold sweat pour out of his body, drenching his clothes. He fell to the ground and lay there groaning with the pain. He lay there for a few minutes without moving, hoping the pain would subside. He then dragged himself slowly to the grassy slope next to the pier. Every motion made the pain worse. He pulled his knees up as high as he could against his chest, his face twisting with the pain, his breath catching as he breathed hard.

"Old Dog," he cried out. "Where are you?"

He reached out several times but couldn't find the dog.

"Old Dog," he whispered hoarsely. "Do you hear me, Old Dog?"

He lay there with his eyes shut tight, with colors forming and reforming, and he saw old Pete lying dead among the leaves.

* * * *

Then he was standing at the edge of a great forest, totally motionless, watching the snow come down. It was already thick on the ground, covering up the tracks he had made. Everything seemed terribly quiet, the wind having gone, leaving behind a silence that fell and covered every bit of the ground along with the snow. He looked around and there was nothing but trees, snow, and a dark, brooding sky. He felt slightly appalled by the heavy silence and the snow that fell so quickly. He continued to look about, turning slowly. He couldn't see the dog anywhere. If he had come this way, his tracks were already covered up by the snow.

He leaned his gun against a tree and cupped his gloved hands around his mouth, letting out a long, low whistle that ended with a quick succession of high notes. The sound did not seem to carry and there was no answering bark. He stood there at the edge of the woods and waited, watching the snow curl down like an endless perforated curtain. Everything was changing right before his eyes. He looked back to the point where he had crossed the stream. The field dipped sharply there and he saw the edge of the water crusted with ice and the trees already white. The sky was getting blacker and appeared to be pressing down on the tops of the trees. And everywhere, this terrible silence, this terrible loneliness, this terrible whiteness surrounded him. He couldn't even hear the sound of the brook.

He had been on the other side of the stream when he first noticed the dog wasn't with him anymore. He whistled several times, trying to see through the thick screen of snow. Then he saw a quick movement at the edge of the woods and he walked along the stream until he reached a spot he could cross. By the time he got to the trees, there was nothing.

He stood there now, looking around, but it was impossible to see more than a few yards and every minute it was getting worse. His legs felt tired and ached very badly. Finally he loosened his jacket and took off his scarf. He spread it out smooth on the snow, knowing that the dog would stay there if he smelled it before the snow had a chance to cover it up.

He took one last look around and felt again the vast white silence.

He picked up his gun then and went into the darkness of the woods. He knew Pete would be there.

LESSONS TO BE LEARNED

The old man described here was at the end of the trail, suffering from emphysema and arteriosclerosis. He has Cheyne-Stokes respirations during which breathing actually ceases for a short while during sleep, a not uncommon finding in the aged. But he was suffering more intensely from the relationship he had with his daughter-in-law and son. Being alone in his own home and faced with the increasing debilities of old age, he invited them to live with him. Frequently, in such situations, the elderly individual soon becomes a stranger in his own home. He is held hostage by old age and his own relatives. The old man, like many others, finds the doctor too busy to spend much time with him. In this situation, a family discussion would have been helpful. It's doubtful that any kind of talking would have changed the daughter-in-law to any significant degree. But the bonding with the doctor would have been stronger and the old man would have been willing to come out of his protective shell and reveal his miseries more readily. And the stronger the bond, the more apt is the patient to take his medications according to the directions given him.

Fortunately, the old man had a dog to talk to, a friend forever loyal and forgiving, just like the old cabbie and his horse in the famous story by Anton Chekhov. He had already lost his old buddy, Pete, who had helped to make his life worth living. After Pete's death, loneliness rests at the old man's elbow like a vulture waiting for him to die.

The doctor apparently didn't take the time to understand that many old people don't fear death. They actually welcome it. Death to them is not depressing. It's living that's depressing. But the old man wants death to come the same way it happened to his friend Pete, while hunting.

PATIENT BEWARE—

After the old man's discussion with his son, he finally realizes there is only one avenue of escape for him and his dog. A terminal hallucination allows him to take that route peacefully and naturally.

Chapter Twenty-one

A Lady-in-Waiting

"Well, Miriam, you did it again," I said.

Miriam sat primly by the desk in the examining room, looking sweet and innocent.

"What did I do, Doctor?" she said.

"Don't look so pure and holy, Miriam," I said. "You've been eating chocolates again and your blood sugar is now six hundred."

"Oh my goodness," she said. "I suppose that's high."

"Your goodness had nothing to do with it. It's the devil in you."

"So what do we do now, Doctor?"

"This time you've broken all your old records and your sugar is high enough to put you into the hospital and start insulin," I said.

"I was afraid you were going to say that, Doctor. I've had so many problems lately and I've been so upset."

"I thought you were leading a well-controlled, organized, active existence, Miriam. What happened?"

"Well, I was, Doctor," Miriam said. "I've been very active in the church, as you know. I'm in charge of arranging all the flowers on the altar every Saturday and Sunday. I pass the collection basket at every service. I count all the money and make out the bank deposit slips. We recently published a parish cookbook which you were nice enough to buy. As you can see, I've been very busy and happy with what I'm doing."

"What's bothering you then?"

"My son, Mathew, has come to live with me and my life is just no longer the same. I hate to say this about my son, but he's completely worthless. He's on welfare and hasn't worked a day since Jeannine, his wife, divorced him. He doesn't pay child support and drinks like a fish. Ever since he moved into my house, I've been a slave. I have to do his laundry and cook for him. He's always borrowing money from me. I even had to ask one of my neighbors to drive me down to your office because he's got my car. My life has become pure hell."

She started to cry.

"You know, of course, Miriam, that your emotions have a significant impact on your diabetes, and that it's very difficult to control your blood sugar if you're under a constant emotional strain. I'll admit you to the hospital for a few days. You'll be able to get a good rest and perhaps think of ways to solve some of your personal problems. During that time, you'll learn to give yourself insulin. We'll stabilize your sugar and when you finally leave the hospital, you'll feel like a new woman."

"Here I am, seventy-five-years old and still facing all these problems with my son," she said. "Wouldn't it be nice to be able to divorce your children and say to them, 'I'm no longer your mother. Please go torment somebody else.'"

"You must understand, Miriam, that part of the problem is your own doing," I said.

"In what way, Doctor?"

"You haven't been firm enough with your son. You know what happens to women who don't know how to say 'No.' As long as you keep handing him money, he's going to keep his hand out for more. He has taken over your car because you have allowed him to do just that. He has enslaved you because you've permitted this to happen. I have another lady very much like you. Her son is an attorney who has his own law firm in Hartford with three other attorneys working for him. Last week, she told me her son borrowed one hundred thousand dollars from her because business was bad."

"That's a lot of money," Miriam said.

"That exactly half of all the money she has," I said. "I asked her what kind of car her son drives. 'A Mercedes,' she answered. 'And your daughter-in-law, what kind does she drive?' 'A BMW,' she answered. I told her she was subsidizing her son's extravagant life style, what was called 'conspicuous consumption' years ago and is now recognized as 'yuppie extravagance.' All you have to learn to say is one simple word: 'No.' Do you think for one minute they would help you if you were in dire need?"

"No, I don't think my son would. But of course, he's in no position to help anyone. It's so hard to say 'No' to your own flesh and blood."

"If you keep giving, Miriam, your son will keep taking. Next in importance to your good health, Miriam, is your economic independence. Those are the two most valuable treasures you must guard jealously as you live through old age. Many older people today, are turning over all their assets to their children to avoid taxes. Then when they enter convalescent hospitals, they are admitted as welfare recipients. That is a very foolish thing to do."

"I'm sure my son would make my life even more miserable if I suddenly told him to get out. I think it would be easier for everybody if I just dropped dead."

"That doesn't sound like the Miriam I know," I said. "You'll feel better after you get out of the hospital and your sugar is down. You know that a high blood sugar can make you feel like an old lady."

"Well, that's what I am," Miriam said.

"Only if you want to be, Miriam. During the seventy-five years you've been on this earth, you have solved bigger problems than this. I remember when you got rid of your drunken husband."

"Yes, and now he has come back to haunt me in the shape of my son."

I admitted Miriam to the hospital at two o'clock and left orders for her, including the basic diabetic diet, insulin and laboratory work. I also left instructions to repeat the blood sugar in four hours and to call me at that time with the results.

Six o'clock came and went and there was no call from the hospital. I called the floor and asked for the laboratory results.

"Just a moment, Doctor," the floor nurse said. It seemed a long time before she came back to the phone.

"I'm sorry, Doctor," she said, "but we forgot to notify the lab to draw her blood."

"You what?" I said. I was astonished. "How much insulin has she received since she was admitted?"

There was a long pause.

"I'm sorry to have to tell you this, Doctor, but she hasn't received any. The nurse assigned to her just happened to overlook your patient completely."

"Her blood sugar was six hundred this afternoon in my office. I haven't heard of anything this negligent in all my years in medicine. This, young lady, is rotten medical care. Please have an incident report ready for me to sign in the morning."

I left new orders for blood sugars and insulin and made it very clear that I was to be called in four hours. There was no message for me four hours later, so I called the hospital.

"What is the blood sugar on my patient," I asked the nurse.

"Just a moment," the nurse said.

It was a long time before she came back to the phone, at least five minutes that seemed more like thirty. It wasn't the same nurse that had answered the phone.

"Doctor?"

"Yes," I said.

"I'm really sorry to have to tell you this, but your patient didn't receive any insulin and no blood sugar was done," the nurse said.

"All right," I said, trying to restrain my anger. "I'll give you exactly twenty minutes to get my patient off that floor. Transfer her immediately to another medical floor. I expect to hear from the head nurse on the new floor within the next twenty minutes, asking for new orders. At the same time, have the night nursing supervisor call me immediately."

When the supervisor called back a few minutes later, I explained to her what had happened.

"Now I want you to go to that floor and find out what the problem is. If anything happens to my patient because of this negligence, I'm sure her son will sue the hospital for an astronomical sum. I have never seen such poor medical care in any hospital I've ever been in. It's your job to see this never happens again."

During the night, Miriam's blood sugar gradually came down with insulin. It had spiked to eight hundred during the time she hadn't received any insulin. It was down to one hundred forty by six in the morning. I filled out an incident report, but never heard about it after that. This was not unusual in our hospital. Apparently, filling out an incident report was merely a way to allow the doctor to let off steam. No action was usually taken. The night nursing supervisor called me later and said the whole affair was just a simple oversight.

I reported the matter to the Chief of the Medical Department. He promised that he would look into the problem.

The next day, I saw him in the coffee shop.

"Did you look into that problem I told you about yesterday?" I said.

"Yes," he said, "and I really can't explain how the nurses managed to overlook your patient for eight straight hours. Did you answer your messages immediately?"

"I never got any messages," I said.

"Have you ever done anything to antagonize the nurses on that floor in any way?"

"No," I said, "I haven't. And what difference would that make? Nurses are supposed to be professionals. They cannot show any animosity to the patient merely because they may dislike the physician. That would be unethical. Furthermore, I bend over backwards to be nice to all the nurses, even the ones who have demonstrated repeatedly that they shouldn't have gone into nursing. This time I was so upset, I told them I wouldn't allow any of my patients to be admitted to that specific floor ever again."

"Yes," he said, "I know. They told me they don't want your patients there, either. They're only human, you know."

"Are you the Chief of the Medical Department at this hospital, supposedly dedicated to uphold a high standard of medical care, or are you just another hospital employee hired to defend and make excuses for poor nursing care? If a physician was responsible for such a grievous oversight, you would already have threatened him with loss of his privileges and raised holy hell. I expect you to do your job or I will discuss your performance at the next medical meeting and report you to the Executive Committee."

That specific floor, where the nurses managed to overlook Miriam for eight hours, continued to be the worst floor in the hospital. I checked with several other physicians and they, too, had refused to have their patients admitted there. And that was the way the situation remained for many years.

As for Miriam, her blood sugar stabilized on twenty units of long-acting insulin. She felt much better and her vision improved, as I had expected. She stayed away from the chocolates most of the time. She learned quickly to give herself an extra five to ten units of insulin when the evil urges to eat the forbidden foods overtook her. However, she was never able to say "No" to her son. He went through her bank account like a broker selling junk bonds to a senile politician. Over a six-month period, Miriam gradually gave up her church activities and finally refused to leave the house altogether. She stopped bathing herself, wore the same dress every day, and stopped combing her hair. She had been extremely proud of her coiffure.

I arranged for the public health nurse to come to see her periodically. About every six weeks I'd make a house call to check her progress.

"What's happening to you, Miriam?" I said one day. "You used to be so proud of the way you dressed and took such good care of yourself. And you were so meticulous about the way you took care of your hair. Now look at you."

"You're right, Doctor. I look a bloody mess and I haven't been to church in six months. But you know, I'm a lady-in-waiting."

She looked at me, slyly cocking her head to one side, and then winked.

"What are you waiting for, Miriam?" I said. "Or for whom are you in-waiting?"

"You know what I'm waiting for, Doctor. You're smart enough to know that. After all, we've been going together a long time. And I don't want any of your fancy pills to take while I'm waiting. I'll take my insulin and that's enough. You won't even find one chocolate in the house. I'll just continue to wait peacefully and quietly."

Miriam didn't have to wait long. One week later, she died in her sleep.

LESSONS TO BE LEARNED

As you can see, hospital personnel don't always carry out specific orders properly. Having the Chief of Medicine explain their negligence by saying, "they're only human," is inexcusable and opens the door for more negligence. The physician must be aware that hospital nurses and assistants in his own office can create many problems that can wreak havoc with a patient's care.

But the big problem that was a severe obstacle to the patient's well being was the presence in her home of a useless son, in this case an alcoholic, who was gradually draining the patient of her will to live. So the treatment of a diabetic is more than just diet, insulin or oral medication, and physical activity. It is the physician's duty to probe more deeply and try to understand the personal relationships of the patient to help him in the total care of the individual.

In this case, Miriam became depressed and prayed for death to relieve her of her miseries. It wasn't long before she was granted her wish.

Chapter Twenty-two

My Oldest Brother

"Your brother just had a heart attack."

It was my sister-in-law on the phone.

"He's in the hospital in Springfield. The doctor has just seen him and they're giving him oxygen now. Apparently, he had some water in his lungs."

My brother Stan was the first-born in the family and I was the tenth, following him twenty years later. I always kidded him about our age difference. I told him that up to the age of twelve, I thought he was my father. In spite of the difference in years, we were the closest of the five brothers in the family. He was my father, brother, teacher, confidant, and general navigator through life's tumultuous seas. Two weeks before he turned thirty-seven, he was drafted into the infantry as a rifleman and we were separated for the first time since he graduated from Dartmouth when I was eight. One year later, I quit high school in the middle of my senior year, and joined the infantry myself. Stan had four months of basic training and then was shipped off to Italy where he found himself attacking a company of Germans entrenched on a mountain. He was one of a hundred men thrown into battle against the Germans that day. They captured the mountain by nightfall losing ninety men in the process. All the Germans were dead. Stan suffered a shattered left arm from shrapnel and spent the next six months in the hospital undergoing a series of operations to restore the function of his arm. He was finally discharged with a Purple Heart on his chest and went into teaching.

As I stood listening to my sister-in-law on the phone, I practically ceased to function as a viable human being. I was shaking all over.

When my sister-in-law went to work that morning, my brother had told her that he wasn't feeling well and was planning to stay home from school. He taught at the A.D. Higgins Junior High School in Enfield, the same school where I had attended seventh and eight grades. After she had left for work, he called his doctor who came down to the house around nine. Stan had developed a very labile form of diabetes mellitus type II after his discharge from the army, which was difficult to control even with insulin. He always had wide swings in his blood-sugar levels. The doctor, knowing his diabetic history, didn't bother with any further questioning regarding his symptomatology, nor did he perform a physical examination. He merely checked his urine with a dip stick and told Stan that his diabetes was out of control.

"You have diabetic acidosis and I'm going to have you admitted to the hospital in Springfield," the doctor had said. "I'll call a specialist to handle your case."

He then advised my brother to make his own arrangements to get to the hospital. It wasn't until four in the afternoon that Stan was finally able to get in touch with my brother-in-law, who promised to take him there around six-thirty. By the time they arrived at the hospital, Stan was unable to walk or breathe properly. His lips were blue and he was breathing very rapidly.

He was given oxygen immediately and felt greatly relieved.

"This is the first decent breath I've been able to take all day," he said.

The EKG revealed an anterior myocardial infarction, a heart attack involving the major artery supplying blood to the left ventricle, the main pumping chamber of the heart. The heart was too weak to pump the blood normally and fluid was beginning to leak out into the lungs.

That was when my sister-in-law came to the phone and called me.

While she was telling me the various details, the doctor gave my brother an intravenous injection of Cedalanid, a rapid-acting digitalis preparation.

"Just a minute," she said. "Everybody is rushing back into Stan's room. Hang on. I'll be right back."

It was only ten minutes before she came back on the phone, but it seemed an eternity.

"Stan just died," she said.

I was already crying. It was a well-known fact that an intravenous injection of Cedalanid can cause cardiac arrest when administered during the acute phase of a myocardial infarction.

He was fifty-two and here it is thirty-seven years later and I can honestly state that I have never recovered from the shock of that day.

LESSONS TO BE LEARNED

When my brother, Stan, suffered his heart attack, the most prominent symptoms were weakness and dyspnea (shortness of breath). The doctor didn't bother to take any history because my brother had been under his care many years for his diabetes. That was mistake number one. If the doctor had bothered to question my brother closely, he would have elicited a history of heaviness in the mid-chest area. Some patients don't describe this as pain. In his haste, the doctor bypassed any further history-taking and jumped to the conclusion that Stan's labile diabetes was the problem. Mistake number two. He then proceeded to check the urine for sugar and found it to be very high. Under the stress of a fresh myocardial infarction in a diabetic the sugar rises precipitously. The doctor concluded that my brother's diabetes was out of control.

The big mistake here was not the fact that the physician made a wrong diagnosis, but that he failed to realize his patient was gravely ill. The least we can expect from a competent physician is the recognition of a life-threatening illness.

My brother was severely out of breath and yet he was told to make his own arrangements to get to the hospital that was eight miles away. He didn't get there for at least 9-10 hours. By then he was in severe congestive heart failure and had runs of irregular cardiac rhythm.

The specialist chose to give him Cedalanid intravenously, which is contraindicated in a severe myocardial infarction because the heart is irritable and extremely sensitive and can progress quickly to a deadly irreversible ventricular fibrillation, followed by cardiac arrest and death. And that's exactly what happened.

PATIENT BEWARE—

Cedalanid is one of a group of cardiac drugs called cardiac glycosides. These drugs have a powerful effect on the heart. They increase the force of myocardial contraction and also increase the refractory period of the atrio-ventricular node, thereby inhibiting runs of irregular rhythm, such as premature contractions. These drugs also affect the sinoatrial node through the sympathetic and parasympathetic nervous systems. These nodes are specialized clusters of cardiac cells that initiate and control the beating of the heart through a network of beaded cardiac fibers called Purkinje's fibers (named after Johannes Evangelista Purkinje, a Bohemian physiologist who first identified them).

An acute myocardial infarction associated with severe cardiac failure which causes fluid to fill the lungs due to back pressure in the venous-arterial system makes the patient extremely sensitive to these drugs.

At a medical meeting devoted to cardiac arrhythmias, attended by many cardiologists, I happened to mention during a break that an internationally known cardiologist had recently given a talk on this same subject, stating that cardiologists kill more patients than they ever save by using antiarrhythmic drugs. All the cardiologists poohpoohed that statement, saying it was a gross exaggeration. Two weeks later, the Federal Drug Administration withdrew an antiarrhythmic drug because its use caused a 200% increase in cardiac mortality.

Chapter Twenty-three

My Second Oldest Brother

About two years after Stan's death my brother Walt called me one night and told me that his hemorrhoids were bleeding. I checked him the next day and did a rectal exam. He had both internal and external hemorrhoids. The internal hemorrhoids were bleeding. It seemed to be a simple problem.

"Medicine is full of red herrings," I told him. "You can have bleeding hemorrhoids that we can see easily, and about twelve inches above, beyond the reach of my finger, a cancerous mass can be silently growing without any significant symptoms until it's too late to save you."

"I know you're leading up to something that isn't going to be pleasant," my brother said.

"You're right," I said. "Just to be on the safe side, I'm going to refer you for a sigmoidoscopy. The doctor will insert a tube into your rectum and lower colon just to make sure you don't have a cancer growing there. If that's negative, I'll order a barium x-ray of your colon. And if that's also negative, we'll go out and have a great dinner somewhere."

Unfortunately, at sigmoidoscopy, a malignant mass was found in the colon approximately sixteen centimeters from the anal ring. He was referred by the gastroenterologist to the chief of surgery at the city hospital. I got a call from the surgeon the next day. He told me that he had booked my brother for an abdominal-perineal resection, the type of surgery that results in a colostomy.

"Is there any chance of doing a primary resection and saving his rectum," I asked him.

"Impossible," he said quickly. "The lesion is too low."

I didn't accept that as a final answer. I called Dr. Mosenthal at the Dartmouth-Hitchcock Medical Center where I had taken my residency in Hanover, New Hampshire.

"I'm doing primary resections far lower than sixteen centimeters with excellent results," he said.

I then called a friend of mine, Dr. Andrew Canzonetti, a surgeon in New Britain, whom I admired not only as a friend, but as a highly skilled surgeon. I asked his opinion.

"Technically, it certainly is more difficult than an abdominalperineal, but it's worth doing and of course, the quality of life is vastly improved for the patient. Many of the older surgeons weren't trained in low resection and prefer to do abdominal-perineal resections with a colostomy."

"Will you do it for Walt, Andy?" I said.

"You know I will, Ed," he said.

I had my brother transferred to The New Britain General Hospital, where Dr. Canzonetti was on staff. When the city hospital surgical resident found out about the transfer, he exploded.

"Your brother, by transferring you to that smaller hospital, is practically signing your death certificate," he told my brother in disgust.

Walt fainted in my arms as he told me about the resident's reaction. We had been walking down the hall of the city hospital the night before the transfer. I caught him just before he hit the floor. I stretched him out on the floor and waited for him to come to. Patients and visitors were walking by, looking at us oddly. Nobody offered to help.

Three days later, my brother had his surgery at The New Britain General Hospital. Dr. Canzonetti had Dr. George Bray assist him. They completed a primary resection of the cancerous mass without any unusual difficulty. No colostomy was necessary. Three lymph nodes outside the colon were positive for cancer. I never told my brother about this. He recovered nicely from his operation. I expected him to die from his malignancy in one or two years. He lived twenty-four years after his cancer was excised. No chemotherapy was ever given.

About one month after my brother's cancer surgery, I read an interesting medical article that concluded that patients who have operations for colon cancer and have warts excised at approximately the same time, survive a much longer period of time than patients who don't have warts removed. This sounded almost impossible to believe. It was not just anecdotal information, but a study of three hundred patients. I asked my brother if he had any warts. He told me he had one on his ankle. I excised it immediately. Apparently, excision of the warts stimulates the immune system.

I'm sure there are many disbelievers out there, especially among the doctors. But let them explain how my brother survived twenty-four years with three positive lymph nodes. I was willing to try anything that could prolong his survival. There is no doubt that the excision of his cancer by competent surgeons and the resultant stimulation of the immune system that occurs in some patients were the reasons for his survival.

Sixteen years later, at the age of sixty-four and with all of his parts still intact, Walt walked into the emergency room of a hospital in South Carolina complaining of the "flu." He had been superintendent of the Bigelow Sanford Carpet Company in Enfield, and when the company abandoned its operations there, he was transferred to South Carolina as superintendent of its Eastern Seaboard Distribution Center.

Walt had not felt well all day. His stomach was churning and he felt a moderate dull pain in the upper part of his abdomen.

The doctor in the emergency room was very thorough. He examined my brother and then ordered a chest x-ray, EKG, and a battery of blood tests. The doctor came back in thirty minutes and told him he had the stomach "flu." He then handed my brother a prescription and reassured him he would be all better in two or three days.

During the night, my brother's condition worsened. He stayed awake all night and was glad to see the first light of day. He called his own doctor and was told to come right down. An EKG revealed an acute anterior myocardial infarction. The heart had been weakened by this attack and the doctor heard rales at both bases of Walt's lungs, indicating congestive heart failure.

PATIENT BEWARE—

He was quickly admitted to the hospital by ambulance. Five minutes after his admission, he developed a deadly ventricular arrhythmia and had to be shocked with a defibrillator. A normal rhythm was restored immediately. If this had happened at home, he would have died. His doctor told him later that he had checked the EKG and the chest x-ray that had been done in the emergency room the night before. That EKG revealed the same changes as the one in the doctor's office the next morning. The chest film showed fluid in both lungs.

The doctor told Walt that a time study had been done on radiologists to determine the average length of time spent reading a chest film. It was ten seconds, about the same length of time spent looking at the check received in payment for reading the x-ray. An emergency room physician spends more time but usually knows less about what he's viewing.

My brother subsequently made an uneventful recovery. Eight years later, while reading the newspaper, he slumped over dead. He was seventy-two years old.

Walt was the one who taught me to love music and encouraged me to play the violin. He also taught me French, geometry, algebra, and how to behave properly. He was a strict authoritarian.

It is unfortunate that most men don't have brothers like the ones I had.

LESSONS TO BE LEARNED

Many older surgeons were trained in doing abdominal-perineal resections for cancer of the lower descending colon because it was not only easier to do technically, but also the belief at that time was that the cancer could metastasize downward, when actually it metastasizes upward. It therefore is unnecessary to remove all of the surrounding tissue beyond the safe zone including the rectum and leave the patient with a colostomy. Today, newer types of medical treatment actually prolong the lives of patients with this type of cancer. But 35 years ago, the chemotherapy that was given for cancer of the colon was absolutely useless and probably did more harm than good because of its deleterious effect on the patient's immune system.

As for my brother's initial visit to the emergency room where he was told he had the "flu" when he was actually suffering from an acute myocardial infarction, this was inexcusable. I would hate to make a list of all the serious mistakes committed in the emergency rooms of the hospitals in this country. Yet the good work that is done far outweighs the bad.

But the fact remains, if a patient goes to a typical city hospital emergency room after midnight, he is immediately in the center of bedlam, a medical no man's land. He is lost among the derelicts, the homeless, the drug addicts, the knife wounds, the gunshot wounds, the automobile accidents, the people who don't have insurance, and the patients who don't bother to have private physicians. In many city hospitals, over 50% of the E.R. visits are drug related. Just by calling his own private physician before going to the emergency room, the patient can avoid most of this confusion. If the E.R. physician knows that he has to call a private attending doctor regarding the patient's condition, fewer mistakes are made because in that case two physicians are involved and the private physician usually knows whether he can depend on the E.R. doctor's diagnostic acumen.

In my brother's case, the EKG and the chest x-ray were both misinterpreted. It was pure luck that he survived the night and was in the hospital when he developed his deadly arrhythmia and had to be shocked.

There is no substitute for a patient's own physician.

Chapter Twenty-four

The Old Man and the Mountain

As he sat there eating the ice cream cone I had just handed him through the car window, he began to laugh like a child with a new toy. He took bigger and bigger bites until he started to cough and choke. Ice cream flew in all directions, splattering the windshield in front of him as he continued to laugh and choke and swallow all at the same time. It was so hot in the car that within a few minutes the ice cream began to melt and drip down his bony fingers.

"Those doctors at the Mary Hitchcock are fantastic," he said in a thick, rasping voice in between mouthfuls of ice cream. "Just a few years ago I was taking ninety units of insulin every day and they wouldn't let me eat anything I liked."

He laughed louder as the mixture of spittle and ice cream dripped down his chin onto his heavy woolen overcoat, his eyes fierce and glaring one moment and glazed and wandering the next.

"Now," he said, "I can eat everything I want and I don't have to take insulin anymore."

His eyes clouded over and his face suddenly twisted into a mask of anguish.

"But everything tastes the same, goddammit. Insipid, absolutely insipid."

With that, he threw the remains of his ice cream cone out the window and spat at the same time, the globoid mixture of saliva and ice cream barely missing me as I executed a rapid, intricate maneuver that would have put a bullfighter to shame.

He closed the window of the car with some effort and huddled in his heavy overcoat, the ice cream having made him chilly. His beak-like nose protruded from below the visor of his woolen cap, making him look like some monstrous bird that had been covered up by some cruel individual with an unusual sense of humor.

"Time to go, boy," he muttered into his scarf.

It was just one hour before that I had helped him dress for this ride. The temperature was ninety degrees with the sun bright and hot, but the Colonel had insisted on wearing long underwear, a heavy woolen shirt, an English tweed suit, and a long, heavy winter over-coat.

"Are you sure you're not going to be too hot, Colonel?" I had said, as I maneuvered him into the car back at the base camp.

"Yes, yes, yes," the Colonel had said impatiently. "Don't you think I know how to dress for this climate?"

As I was about to slide behind the wheel, the Colonel added, "Better put the heater on and don't forget to close your window."

I had visions of collapsing from heat stroke, so I ran back to the cabin and put on my bathing suit and sneakers. The Colonel didn't even glance at me as I slid into the driver's seat. Off we went on our excursion, a New Hampshire version of the odd couple.

My glasses kept fogging up and the sweat poured down my back and dripped off my elbows. Except for a few astonished stares from tourists, the trip was otherwise uneventful.

It was July 1951, and these were the last living remains of Colonel Henry Teague, owner of the Mount Washington Cog Rail-road. He was ravaged by diabetes that had been miraculously "cured" but left him dangling at the end of a seventy-eight year old rope that looked more and more like a hangman's noose. He was an odd collection of old arthritic bones, arteriosclerotic blood vessels, and a flabby heart, all powered by a demented, paranoid brain that slipped rapidly into and out of reality. His face was gaunt with the skin pulled tight across the bones, his sunken eyes at once fierce and savage, but more often vacant and wandering, the sorrowful owner of taste buds that were incapable of performing their assigned task of tasting.

One month earlier, Dr. Syvertsen, the Dean of Dartmouth Medical School, had sighted me over the top of his glasses while I was washing a mountain of dirty trays and dishes in the Mary Hitchcock Memorial Hospital cafeteria.

"This summer you will be the Colonel's boy, Doctor," the Dean had said.

Among his many other duties, Dr. Syvertsen also ran an unofficial employment agency, managing it like a general deploying his troops. We called him the "Great White Father." There were no ifs, ands, or buts to his decisions. Every summer a Dartmouth man was chosen to be the Colonel's boy. That summer, destiny in the form of Dean Syvertsen, had chosen me.

Within a few weeks, I was up in Whitefield, New Hampshire, sitting next to Colonel Teague who was lying in a freshly-made bed in the Whitefield Hospital, looking like a corpse that was ready to be taken to the morgue. He had just been brought up from Dick's House at Dartmouth, still overwhelmed by his new freedom from his old slave-master insulin.

The Colonel would lie in bed, his face a harsh and forbidding mask of sculptured putty, hands folded across his chest, breathing noisily. I read the daily newspapers to him as he drifted off to sleep. He would awake suddenly with a snort, a gurgle, and a paroxysm of coughing, as he aspirated some of the sticky mucus that lay in the back of his throat, sequestered like a tenacious, poisonous mucoid globule waiting to plug up his trachea.

His rhythmical breathing would gradually slow down and then periodically stop. I would cock an ear and watch his chest and wait. I remember holding my own breath as I waited for the Colonel to start breathing again. This was typical of Cheyne-Stokes breathing, a waxing and waning of respiration seen in the elderly and individuals with head injuries.

One day while he wandered in and out of a semi-stupor, lying there peacefully in bed after a sumptuous meal which he described as "totally without savor," I too must have dozed off, but a sudden ear-splitting shriek from the Colonel made me leap from the chair. His thin bony fingers clawed the air in front of him. Saliva flew in a fine spray from his mouth. His eyes glared fiercely as he desperately tried to say something, but his tongue refused to obey his garbled command.

I ran out into the hallway for the nurse assigned to him but she had gone to dinner and the bare white walls were almost a shock to see. Back in the room, the Colonel was still in a spasm of silence, fingers still clawing the air, a look of extreme agony on his face. He seemed to be staring at the corner of the room where the bedpan reposed in its icy silvery splendor. Not knowing what else to do, and having made a rapid interpretation of the Colonel's seizure, I grabbed the bedpan, flung aside the bed covers, and with one swift motion slipped the pan under his scrawny buttocks.

The Colonel's silent seizure ended with a howl heard from one end of the hospital to the other. He shot off the bedpan as if propelled by some mysterious force, landing at the foot of the bed in a heap.

"You son-of-a-bitch," the Colonel finally exploded, the words piercing the air like shells from a 155mm howitzer. "Boy, you son-of-a-bitch," he repeated, this time more slowly and deliberately, enjoying each word as if he could taste it. "Do you know what your main function in life is?"

The question caught me by surprise. Here I thought he was experiencing his last agonizing twitch on this earth and suddenly we were in a philosophical discussion.

"No," I answered. "I hadn't thought much about my main function in life since I left the army, Colonel."

"Well, I will tell you, boy," the Colonel said. "Your main function in life is to make sure my goddamned bedpan is warm before you slip it under my skinny old ass. You can kill an old man like me by simply doing what you just did."

I can just imagine a death certificate with that on it, I thought to myself. By then, three or four nurses, responding to the Colonel's death yell, had entered the room. I made a hasty retreat as I heard the Colonel telling them, "That young son-of-a-bitch tried to kill me."

The nurses told me later that the Colonel was constipated for two weeks after that episode. He also took great pleasure in recounting his recurrent nightmare in which I tried to beat him to death with a bedpan.

As the weeks passed, the Colonel was getting increasingly excited about returning home to his mountain. Colonel Arthur Teague, his unofficially adopted son, was busy getting the cabin ready at the base camp. He would have preferred keeping the old Colonel at

Whitefield because of all the other activities associated with starting the new season. But the old man insisted on going home, probably realizing that this was the last summer that he could enjoy the mountain.

The old Colonel gradually took me into his confidence as he forgot the bedpan incident. He told me how he had bought the Mount Washington Cog Railroad, including the base camp, the entire top of the mountain, and a permanent right of way from the Boston and Maine Railroad during the Great Depression for a few thousand dollars.

"A paltry sum," he would say in his rasping voice, indicating that the B&M officials should have had their heads examined.

He spoke about getting his honorary title of Colonel bestowed by the governor of New Hampshire and his chance meeting with Arthur Teague, who had been a real colonel in the U.S. Army. The old Colonel had talked Arthur into coming back to the mountain to help him run the cog railroad. Both their names being Teague was a mere coincidence.

At the beginning, their relationship was excellent. But as the old Colonel grew older, his dementia was an increasing strain on Arthur.

"Boy, be careful," the old Colonel would say, whispering as though confiding a secret. "He's trying to kill me."

His eyes would dart furtively, searching the room.

"Who's trying to kill you, Colonel?"

"Haven't you been listening, boy?" he'd say angrily, his eyes furious for a moment, his face sly and malicious. "Arthur, of course. Don't you see what's going on? He's been trying to kill me for years. He wants my money but he's not going to get it. I fooled him and I'm still alive."

Then he would drift off into left field, his mind wandering aimlessly among the events of his past, constantly rearranging the bits and pieces of his life and trying vainly to perceive some purpose and coherence among the disjointed fragments, finally surrendering completely to the half-remembered ghosts that continued to haunt him.

The Colonel's cabin at the base camp was about one-half mile from the cog railroad ticket office. The living room was made over into a bedroom and a large swath had been cut through the woods opposite the large windows straight to the ticket office. I would stand there with binoculars and count the number of people in line waiting to buy tickets to go to the top of the mountain.

"How many in line, boy?"

"Ten in line, Colonel, and another six waiting for the next train."

"That's good, boy. That's real fine."

A few minutes would pass and he would start the same routine all over again.

"How many in line, boy?"

Occasionally, when the Colonel was in an especially ugly mood, I would pad the figures and describe dozens of tourists that weren't there. He would then soften up and become somewhat jovial, but it was becoming more difficult to calm his vicious temper.

In the past, Arthur had ropes strung from wall to wall in the Colonel's bedroom. These were used to support the old man when he was still able to walk by himself. This last year, however, he was only able to take a few short steps so I removed the ropes.

My room was upstairs and a loud bell had been installed near the bed. The button activating the bell was always by the Colonel's side day and night. Unfortunately, the Colonel dozed frequently during the day, and stayed awake most of the night, with the result that I began to suffer from lack of sleep. Every hour during the entire night, the Colonel's knobby finger pressed the button. Most of the time it was a long steady ring, but when he was impatient with my arrival, he would play an irritated rhythm, a rat-tat-tat that pounded on my poor sleep-deprived brain like a jackhammer.

Stumbling down the stairs, I would stagger to the Colonel's bed.

"Boy, what took you so long?"

It was the same greeting no matter how quickly I came. I'd mumble something but he'd never bother to listen.

"Never mind, never mind, I don't want to listen to any of your silly excuses, anyway. Adjust my blankets and let me get some sleep."

About one hour later, the bell would ring again. This continued all night. After a week of bell ringing, I was in desperate straits. It was between the bell and me. One of us had to go. It was a matter of survival. Of course, I could have strangled the old man, but I thought of a simpler, more humane solution. I merely mentioned the problem to Arthur.

"A simple problem like that requires a simple solution," Arthur said in a soft understanding voice. "I was wondering how long you could take it before you mentioned the bell. You lasted two days longer than all the rest of the boys."

I followed him to my room. He ripped off the cover of a book of matches and folded it twice. He then inserted the wedge between the hammer and the bell. It seemed that he had done this many times before.

"What if the old man really needs me some night?" I said.

"Do you think at his age it would really make any difference?"

"No, I guess not," I said.

"I'll leave it up to you how often you want to go down and check on him during the night. Once a night should be enough."

The first few nights after the bell had been silenced, I slipped downstairs quietly and listened to the Colonel fuming and fussing with the bell button. The next morning, he greeted me angrily.

"Where were you last night, boy? I pressed that button till I was blue in the face and you didn't come down once."

"You did?" I said, feigning surprise. "That's funny. I slept through the whole night without hearing it once. I'll check it out immediately."

After a few more days, he forgot the whole affair and never mentioned the bell again.

Every morning, my first duties consisted of closing the curtains because the sun shone directly on the Colonel's bed. I would then light the gas radiators beneath the windows.

"I don't like those drapes resting directly on those radiators, Colonel," I said to him one morning. "Some day we're going to have a fire."

"Just do what you're told, boy. You're not paid to think. Close the drapes and go get my breakfast."

All right, you old buzzard, I'd mutter to myself. Someday this whole cabin will go up in smoke and you'll be sorry that you didn't listen to me.

One morning after getting the Colonel's breakfast, I went back to the mess hall and enjoyed a leisurely breakfast myself, staying longer than usual. I strolled casually back to the Colonel's cabin, feeling lazy as I watched the early morning sun slanting through the trees. I was in no great hurry to confront the old tyrant. As I approached the cabin I saw wisps of smoke lazily drifting through the windows. I rushed in and saw the old Colonel sitting on the edge of the bed in a panic. The curtains were smoldering on top of the hot radiators and the room was full of smoke. The Colonel was in a frenzy, jumping up and down, yelling, "Fire, fire, fire. That young son-of-a-bitch is trying to kill me again."

I tore down the curtains and threw them outside. I opened all the windows wide. The room cleared rapidly. When I had finished, I saw the Colonel sitting on the edge of his bed almost smiling. That night he had a great time telling Arthur how I had nearly finished him off.

"You would have been a rich man, Arthur, if that son-of-a-bitch had succeeded in his plot to knock me off."

The next morning, the Colonel did not ask me to light the gas radiators or to close the drapes that were no longer there. That too was forgotten along with the bell that would no longer respond to his frantic pressing.

My last day as the Colonel's boy came rather suddenly about two weeks before our next semester in medical school was scheduled to begin. We were parked in front of the ticket office so that the Colonel could keep count of the people buying tickets. He was dressed in his usual manner, woolen shirt, tweed suit, heavy overcoat and woolen cap pulled down over his ears, his beak-like nose pointing directly at the ticket office.

It was a busy day with crowds of people swarming around buying tickets, waiting for the next train, bustling about the gift shop, and others just strolling around enjoying the beauty of the mountain on a brilliantly clear and sunny day. The car was terribly hot with all the windows up and I sat there in a pool of sweat, eyes closed in a semi-trance, dreaming of cool breezes and cascading ice water. While the Colonel's attention was on the ticket office, I reached out and cranked the window down a few inches. Without turning his head, the Colonel responded immediately.

"I feel a draft, boy. I feel cold air coming in." His voice was somewhat muffled by the scarf around his chin. "Is there a window open in this car?" he continued impatiently.

The old devil had seen me.

"I thought I'd let in some oxygen, Colonel. You looked like you were breathing hard."

"I don't need any extra oxygen, boy. Close the window and keep it closed."

Just then a plump lady came over and stood directly in front of the car, blocking the Colonel's view of the ticket office. He let out a snort and leaning over, depressed the horn. The lady nearly leaped out of her sandals. She turned towards us with a horrified look on her face. She gasped for air and appeared about to faint.

The Colonel was still leaning on the horn, trying to motion her to one side, but the heavy overcoat hindered his movements and he appeared to be twitching in a spasm of agitation.

I stepped out of the car and quickly went over to the lady, fearing she was going to collapse.

"Please accept our apology for frightening you," I said, "but the Colonel lost his balance for a moment and accidentally leaned on the horn."

I looked back at the car. The Colonel was still blowing the horn, his face contorted in anger, a withered old man lost in his heavy overcoat, frantically beating the air with his right hand, listing to the left, and leaning on the horn with all his might.

"Is something wrong with him?" she said, nodding her head toward the Colonel.

It was hard to hear her voice over the blare of the horn.

"He's just an old man," I said softly.

I returned to the car.

The lady walked off, looking back several times with a questioning look on her face. By then, a few other people were beginning to gather around the car, looking inside at the Colonel.

When I opened the door, I heard the Colonel snarling and gasping for air.

"I know what you told her, you son-of-a-bitch. You told her I was crazy, didn't you?"

His hands clutched the air trying to reach me, but his overcoat was too great an impediment, restricting his motions by its sheer weight.

"I'll show you how crazy I am. You're fired, you hear? Get off this mountain and never come back. Crazy, am I? I'll show you who's crazy."

I reached over and removed the car keys and made sure the brakes were set. I shut the door while he was still bellowing like a wild animal and walked down the hill to the base camp.

I only looked back once. I could still see his mouth moving in a silent fury, his clenched fists pummeling the air, a tragic prisoner trapped by his overcoat and senility. A cold wind came down off the mountain and made me shudder. A lone bird chirped in the distance. I looked up at the mountain. It was serene and immutable, protruding from the earth's crust like a giant monument glorifying the earth itself.

That was the last time I saw the Colonel.

I explained the whole affair to Arthur. He was very understanding. He told me I had lasted longer than any of the other Colonel's boys.

The summer was at an end and about six weeks after I left the mountain to go back to school, I heard the old man had died.

If he could have had his last wish, I know that he would be lying there now with his long underwear on, his woolen socks and shirt, his English tweed suit and scarf, and his monstrous winter overcoat, with his woolen cap pulled down over his ears, his nose sticking out like the beak of an eagle.

As for his final resting place, he would have preferred a spot immediately in front of the cog railroad ticket office. Even six feet down, there would be a distinct tremor in the earth as the tourists walked across the site to buy tickets for the ride to the top of the mountain. The earth would move with every train that pulled out.

That way the old man and the mountain would have been united forever. And that would have made the Colonel very happy.

LESSONS TO BE LEARNED

Colonel Henry Teague was a victim of senile dementia. The prevalence of this type of dementia, which by definition, means a deterioration of mental capacity, increases with age. Failure of memory may be the first obvious symptom in dementia, even though all elderly individuals suffer some loss of memory without progressing to dementia. The development of dementia can frequently be so gradual as to go unnoticed except by family members close to the patient. Emotional outbursts often accompany progressive dementia as well as paranoia as seen in this chapter, making it extremely difficult for close relatives living with such patients to maintain the detachment so necessary for proper medical care.

Alzheimer's disease is a form of dementia, one that usually has its beginning in the 5th or 6th decade of life, but can begin later. Years ago, this form of dementia was called "presenile dementia." Alzheimer's, however, has specific changes that occur in the brain, namely neurofibrillary tangles easily seen microscopically at autopsy unrelated to senile dementia. To make matters worse, today it is common to label nearly all intellectual deterioration as Alzheimer's. And to complicate the situation even more, it is becoming increasingly difficult to separate senile dementia and Alzheimer's clinically as the population ages. A recent study of this condition concluded that only two-thirds of cases diagnosed as Alzheimer's are truly Alzheimer's when studied at autopsy.

Colonel Teague also suffered from end-stage diabetes mellitus. He had been a diabetic for many years requiring up to 90 units of insulin daily. How can it be explained that in his last year of life his diabetes was clinically absent? We know that by removing the pituitary, the diabetic condition is ameliorated. Advanced age, by the process of arteriosclerosis and associated microscopic infarctions can also render the pituitary powerless.

Another characteristic of advanced age is the sensation of chilliness experienced by elderly individuals. These patients are very sensitive to heat loss and may die from surprisingly short periods of exposure to winter temperatures. This is why Colonel Teague dressed himself as though he was preparing for arctic weather even in July. Heavily dressed he was comfortable because he had lost the ability to sweat.

Because of his "adopted" son, Arthur Teague, who was practically a saint, the old Colonel was able to spend the last years of his life on the mountain he loved. While there, he was increasingly difficult to handle. It's unfortunate that most physicians during their training have never been sequestered with individuals like this. This problem of senility will grow larger every year as the population ages and society will have to find new ways to manage it without the government rendering the final solution.

Chapter Twenty-five

A Man's Best Friend

"*I*'m having trouble sleeping, Doctor."

Martin Macklin was a heavy-set, middle-aged automobile salesman. He appeared worried.

"How long have you had this problem, Martin?" I said. I hadn't seen him for the last three years. He had gained about twenty pounds and appeared puffy.

"I really can't say, Doctor. It sort of came over me during the past month. Do you think it's the coffee I've been drinking? I drink about six cups a day."

"Did the coffee bother you before?"

"No, it never seemed to, Doctor."

"Tell me, then, exactly what is your problem in sleeping. Are you worried about anything? Are you depressed?"

"Well, I'm worried about this sleeping problem, but I'm not depressed. It's just that when I lie down to go to sleep I get short of breath for about an hour. After that, I have no difficulty sleeping. That seems odd to me."

"Do you have to prop yourself up on pillows?"

"Yes, I do, Doctor. Sometimes it's so bad that I even have to sit up for a few minutes."

"Can you feel your heart beating?"

"Yes, awfully fast, too. It seems like it's going to jump right out of my chest. The beating even goes all the way up into my neck."

Martin touched his neck with his right hand. His head was bobbing slightly.

"Have you had any swelling of your legs?"

"A little. My ankles seem puffy. I gained about ten pounds in the past month. I think it's the salt. I can't stay away from salted nuts and potato chips."

"Do you have any chest pain either at rest or with exercise?"

"Not while I'm resting," he said. "But when I'm too active, I have an uncomfortable feeling in my chest and my left elbow begins to ache."

"Did you have rheumatic fever as a child, Martin?"

"Not that I can remember, Doctor. You mean with swollen joints and being forced to stay in bed? No, nothing like that. I had a lot of sore throats, though."

On physical examination, the blood pressure was one hundred sixty over fifty. This was the third clue to his problem: a slightly elevated systolic blood pressure (the reading as the heart contracts) and a lower than normal diastolic pressure (the pressure in between contractions). The first clue was a slight bobbing of Martin's head as he related his problem. The second clue was the sudden ten pound weight gain the past month. On examination of his neck, there were visible pulsations of his carotid arteries, the main blood vessels carrying blood to his brain. I felt a "water-hammer" pulse in his wrist. This is more difficult to evaluate. It is a pulse with a powerful, sharp uptake followed by a quick collapse. On slight compression of the fingernails, I saw an alternate blushing and blanching in the nail bed with each cardiac cycle.

With my hand held flat against Martin's chest over the left sternal border (the left side of the breast bone), I felt a delicate vibratory sensation caused by the tumultuous flow of the blood through his heart. This is called a "thrill." Remember, one of the definitions of a "thrill" is a "vibration." I could feel a similar sensation over his aorta, jugular veins, and carotid arteries. On palpation of his heart, the apex was displaced to the left, indicating enlargement. The pulse was hyperkinetic (rapid).

On listening to the heart with the stethoscope, the first sound seemed slightly diminished in intensity. The second sound was markedly diminished and nearly completely replaced by a loud, decrescendo murmur that we describe as "blowing." This lasted almost the entire length of time between beats. The murmur was high-pitched and prominent. This was astonishing to me because Martin had no murmurs on his prior physical examinations.

On listening to the base of his lungs, I heard rales on both sides, sounding similar to velcro being slowly pulled apart. There was slight pitting edema of the ankles. My fingers squeezing caused imprints in the puffy skin.

The EKG revealed changes indicating that the left side of his heart was moderately enlarged. This is the left ventricle, the main pumping chamber of the heart. A chest x-ray also confirmed this enlargement.

After the examination was completed, I came back to Martin's room, where he was sitting in a chair with his head low.

"Well, Doctor," he said, looking very sad. "How long have I got to live?"

"Martin, don't look so sad," I said. "You do have a serious problem, but luckily, it's one that we can solve. You have a leaky valve in your heart, called the aortic valve. When the heart pumps the blood into the aorta, which is the major blood vessel leading from the heart, this valve is supposed to close at the end of the pumping action to allow the heart to fill up in preparation for the next beat. Your valve stays open, allowing a portion of the pumped blood to rush back into the heart, causing a loud murmur over your heart that can be heard easily with a stethoscope. So you have this to and fro rush of blood in your heart. This causes the slight bobbing of your head and the flushing and blanching of your fingernails that I checked before. This leaky valve causes an increased strain on your heart, with a resultant thickening of the cardiac muscle in the left ventricle, the main pumping chamber of your heart. Furthermore the pumping action of the heart has been weakened slightly and you now have a small amount of fluid in your lungs and some swelling in your ankles from the back pressure."

Martin and I continued to discuss his problem for about an hour.

"What if I do nothing, Doctor? What if I just let nature take its natural course?"

"First of all, your wife Sarah won't let you do that. The average life expectancy after the onset of symptoms if nothing is done is about seven years. Death will be caused by heart failure or a sudden deadly irregular rhythm. If you undergo surgery, you should be able to lead a completely normal life because the changes in your heart are still reversible. If you wait till the changes become permanent and then decide to have the surgery, the outcome is much less satisfactory and the risk is much greater.''

I scheduled a stat echocardiogram and sent him to a cardiologist in a large medical center. He confirmed the diagnosis by performing a cardiac catheterization and scheduled his surgery for valve replacement with the chief of the department. About two weeks before the surgery was scheduled, Martin came in with his wife for another discussion.

"I just came to talk with you some more, Doctor, because frankly, I'm scared to death about this surgery."

"It's normal to be frightened, Martin, but let me tell you the good news. Your problem has been diagnosed early. You should have an excellent result. I've had two other patients this past year with the same problem, but in a more advanced state. Both have done exceptionally well. If you like, I'll call them up and I'm sure they'd be happy to discuss all aspects of the surgery with you. There is very little disability after the operation and you're going to be amazed at how rapidly you regain your former good health and vigor. I'm sure the surgeon has discussed all of this with you."

"I haven't seen the surgeon, Doctor," he said. "That's what worries me."

"You mean Doctor Stimson has scheduled you for surgery without seeing you?" I said.

"That's right, Doctor," he said. "The cardiologist called him on the phone and got the date of admission to the hospital, but I've never seen the surgeon."

"That is certainly unusual," I said.

"We thought so, too, Doctor," Sarah said. "Then we thought perhaps we should see a surgeon in another hospital, just to give Martin some confidence."

"Good idea," I said, "but remember, this may also confuse you. I'll make two appointments for Martin. One with Dr. Stimson, the Chief of Cardiac Surgery at the medical center where you saw the cardiologist. He has an excellent reputation. I'll also make another appointment with Dr. Stimson's counterpart at a hospital in Boston. You'll take your records with you. While they interview you, you will interview them. And then, you and your wife will have a better idea where you should have your surgery. Remember, both of these surgeons are equal in ability. Your decision will eventually come down to one point: the institution in which you'd prefer to have your surgery."

Both Martin and Sarah liked this arrangement. Martin had both interviews and was equally impressed by both surgeons. After some procrastination, he finally decided to go to Boston.

His damaged aortic valve was replaced with a pig's valve. His surgery was a complete success. He continued to work for a few more years, and after being named the most outstanding automobile salesman in New England for two consecutive years, he retired to a farm in Maine to raise pigs. I see him every summer for his annual physical examination.

He leads a happy and productive life. He has been a great success at raising pigs. He told me he has never eaten ham or pork since he started his pig farm. His pigs usually win all the blue ribbons at the local fairs much to the disgust of all the other pig farmers.

When asked by a local newspaperman the secret to his success as a pig farmer, Martin answered without hesitation: "I understand pigs and pigs understand me. They instinctively know that I don't eat ham or pork. And furthermore, I owe my life to a pig and so they try harder for a blood brother."

LESSONS TO BE LEARNED

A patient calls the office for an appointment and complains of insomnia. Obviously, there is no need to squeeze him in early, so he is given the first available appointment. But when a more detailed history is elicited, an altogether different problem is revealed. One that requires an immediate appointment. And then the patient throws in another red-herring: coffee. But a careful history will bring out the real problem.

At least fifty per cent of the patients with damaged cardiac valves do not have a history of rheumatic fever. In this case, Martin Macklin suffered from aortic insufficiency. The valve leaflets do not close properly, and the pulse wave is pumped forward by the contraction of the heart, and then races backward through the partially open valve, creating a "blowing" murmur. A murmur is a turbulence in the blood flow. The sound with this type of damaged valve is very similar to the sound you make by saying, "shush-h-h."

The big problem that Martin faced was that the first surgeon never had the patient come to the office to have the procedure of valve replacement explained. The surgeon never examined Martin. This was probably an error of omission committed by the office staff. The cardiologist should never have gotten the appointment for surgery himself. Circumventing routine office procedure frequently results in mistakes. Luckily, the patient felt uneasy and consulted his family physician.

It is amazing how much a physician can conclude about a patient's condition from a good history and a thorough physical examination before any expensive procedures are scheduled to confirm the diagnosis. The physician should establish the diagnosis by his own wits, if that is possible, and not depend on expensive investigative procedures to make up for faulty history taking and inadequate physical examinations.

Chapter Twenty-six

The Clot That Wasn't There

"*J*ohnny can't get out of bed."

It was my sister, Ann, calling from Thompsonville. She sounded very upset.

"Why can't he get out of bed?" I said.

"Every time he tries to get up, he starts vomiting."

"Does he feel like vomiting when he's lying down flat?"

"No. Only when he sits up or tries to stand up," she said. "We just got back from a cruise in the Caribbean two days ago and he had no complaints except maybe a little headache that he thought was caused by seasickness."

"I'll be right over, Ann. Keep him in bed flat on his back."

It was Wednesday afternoon, my usual half-day off. I had a million things I had planned to do. Those could wait, I said to myself, as I jumped into the car and drove the thirty-five miles to their home on Prospect Street in Thompsonville. My brother-in-law, John Pastormerlo, was like a brother to me. He married my sister before I was born, so he was in the family before I made my entrance.

When I got there, he looked perfectly well lying flat in bed, reading the newspaper.

"What the hell is going on with me?" he said. "I can't get out of bed without vomiting."

"Show me," I said.

He grabbed a basin that was on the side of the bed. As soon as he reached a sitting position, he vomited. It was projectile, spewing suddenly and rapidly from his mouth as if blasted from a cannon.

"Lie flat, John," I said quickly.

As soon as he stretched out flat, the vomiting stopped, as suddenly as it had started.

"Do you have a headache, John?" I said.

"Off and on, Ed, but probably no more than usual," John said.

"It seems he has been asking for aspirin more often lately," Ann said.

"Did you fall at any time while you were on that cruise to the Caribbean," I said.

"No," John said. "I haven't fallen anywhere for years."

"Have you banged your head lately?" I said.

"Not lately," John said. "You know I have that low ceiling going down my stairs to the cellar. Well, in the past, I must have hit my head a million times going down the stairs, but I can't remember doing it recently."

"Have you noticed any other changes in your general health, John, like fatigue, drowsiness, or general irritability," I said.

"He's been sleeping a lot since he developed this vomiting," Ann said. "And he seems more irritable than usual."

"Well, wouldn't you be if you couldn't get out of bed? And what can you do in bed lying flat on your back? You sleep, that's what you do. I'm not used to staying in bed. I'm beginning to think I've got a serious problem, Ed."

I checked him over completely. There were no abnormalities. His neurological exam was entirely normal except for the fact he had projectile vomiting on assuming the upright position.

When I finished, I sat on the edge of the bed.

"Well," John said, fiddling with the edge of the bed covers. "What the hell kind of bug did I pick up on that boat?"

"John, I think you have a clot on your brain," I said, "and I'm going to call your doctor in Hartford and he'll admit you to the hospital this afternoon. You can't stay home in this condition."

"How can I have a clot on my brain?" John said. "I told you I don't remember hitting my head recently."

"As a person gets older, John, his brain gradually shrinks. As it does, the suspensory system of the brain is stretched. There are blood vessels in this suspensory tissue and it doesn't take much of a blow to make a tiny little blood vessel tear and start bleeding. Only in Hollywood can the hero get whacked on the head and get up immediately and continue as if nothing happened. This kind of slow bleeding and clotting can go on for weeks and even months before the pressure in your skull is great enough to cause symptoms. Your brain can probably tolerate up to two ounces of blood without causing any unusual symptoms. As the bleeding continues intermittently and the clot gets larger than two ounces, then you can develop projectile vomiting, headache, drowsiness, and irritability. This condition will gradually worsen until you become unconscious if we don't do something about it."

"So what are they going to do with me in the hospital?" John said.

"They'll take x-rays of your head, draw some blood for a variety of blood tests, and then you'll be examined by a neurosurgeon. If he agrees with my diagnosis, he'll schedule you for surgery and remove the clot that's pressing on your brain."

"And if he doesn't agree with your diagnosis?" John said.

"Then we have to look for other conditions that can cause these same symptoms," I said. "But I'm sure you have a subdural hematoma. That's the official terminology for your condition."

I called his internist in Hartford and John was admitted that same day.

The next day his doctor, Dr. Westmore, called me.

"The neurosurgeon examined your brother-in-law and reviewed the x-rays. He said that there is absolutely no evidence for a subdural hematoma. The neurological exam is entirely negative. He thinks John probably has a metastatic carcinoma so I've scheduled him for the all-American work-up to see if he has a cancer hidden somewhere. I'll keep you posted."

"What's your opinion?" I said.

"I think John has a subdural hematoma," Dr. Westmore said.

"So do I," I said. "I hope they don't dilly-dally until John slips into a coma. You know how treacherous a subdural can be."

"Well, he's a little better today, so we'll start with x-rays of his gall bladder, then his kidneys, and end up with a G.I. series and a barium enema."

"I'd be much happier if the neurosurgeon ordered a cerebral angiogram and then performed a diagnostic trephination. I'd bet my last dollar that he has a subdural. I hope the surgeon isn't a mule-headed individual that always tries to prove that the primary physician is wrong."

"We'll see," the internist said. "In the meantime, his condition is stable and he's in no danger."

"It's a very awkward situation when you disagree with your consultant," I said. "You'll have to watch John closely and insist that the neurosurgeon operates before John's condition suddenly worsens. You know how quickly that can happen."

Dr. Westmore agreed.

It took two weeks to complete all the studies. During that time, John's condition seemed to be gradually deteriorating. His headaches were more pronounced and constant. He was very irritable when awake, but very drowsy. He slept most of the time. His oral intake was poor and had to be continually supplemented with intravenous fluids.

Finally, at four o'clock in the morning, exactly two weeks after his admission, he went into a deep coma and appeared close to death. The neurosurgeon came in and performed an emergency trephination as a last resort. This is a procedure where burr holes are drilled through the skull. He found huge bilateral hematomas that he evacuated without difficulty.

John's post-operative course was stormy, a classic example of the problems you can expect when evacuation of a subdural hematoma is delayed to this extent. In fact, the survival rate is only ten percent in this type of situation. It is over ninety percent if the surgery is done early. Post-operatively, John developed a fulminating pneumonia. The sputum was so tenacious, a tracheostomy was done. His breathing had to be assisted with a respirator and he was suctioned every fifteen minutes. Massive doses of antibiotics were injected into his withered old body.

He gradually responded, and after eight weeks in the hospital, he was finally discharged to a convalescent hospital. He was too weak to walk. He was totally bedridden and continued to require oxygen through his tracheostomy tube. He lived this way for another five years and then died quietly in his sleep on Christmas eve, 1979.

LESSONS TO BE LEARNED

Here we have another example of a stubborn surgeon who initially entertains the wrong diagnosis. He does this with such emphasis that all other physicians retreat. But careful follow-up and an open mind could have led to the correct diagnosis. The questioning of a good observant nursing staff would have revealed the gradual deterioration of the patient. But how many physicians do that? Very few, unfortunately. How many doctors read the nurses' notes? Again, very few.

It is the attending physician's obligation to put pressure on a hesitant consulting surgeon. When the attending doctor doesn't agree with the consultant, an awkward situation quickly develops, and the patient is usually the one who suffers. This is especially true when an attending physician works with the same consultants all the time. In this case, another consultant should have been called in after a few more days of observation. But we are all guilty of bowing down before a lordly neurosurgeon. The obvious trepidation on the part of the attending physician and the wrong initial diagnosis of the neurosurgeon resulted in an extremely stormy post-operative course. The patient became a permanent invalid attached to tubes and required constant suction. He had a markedly diminished quality of life and suffered a pitiful existence until death released him from his agony.

Chapter Twenty-seven

A Mere Fainting Spell

Big Bill Hutchinson was a large man, standing six feet four inches and weighing two hundred fifty pounds. He had hands the size of catchers' mitts and it seemed odd to see such a big man surrounded by the flowers he loved so much, delicately arranging them into beautiful bouquets. And when it came to flower arrangements, there was none better than Big Bill. When he turned forty-eight, he quit his job in a neighboring city where he worked as a flower arranger and "front desk" sales clerk. Winning the one hundred thousand dollar lottery helped him to decide that opening up his own flower shop was the right thing to do. He bought an old house not far from the center of town and, within one month, had his grand opening. The rest is history. He and his wife were workaholics, toiling seven days a week, and frequently well into the night. They were an instant success. Both of them were expert flower arrangers and the greatest talkers in central Connecticut. They liked flowers and people and that was the secret of their success.

Much of their work consisted of preparing flowers for the local funeral homes. Big Bill saw many of his friends laid out over the years. He'd stand there and take one last look after setting the flowers in their proper places.

"God, doesn't Jabber O'Houlihan look great, George?" he had said inevitably to George Barton, the funeral director he knew best and whose work he admired the most. "How do you manage to get that little smile on his face? That's utterly amazing!"

George Barton was never tired of hearing such praise.

"We call that the 'Mona Lisa' smile," George answered, his hands folded across his ample paunch. "We are very proud of the way we handle the lips of the dear departed. That is the hardest part of the preparation. You won't see that done with such delicate care in any other funeral home in the entire country. That is what we call *real living art.*"

They both stood there admiring the smile.

"When I go, George," Big Bill said, "I want a smile just like the one you put on Jabber O'Houlihan. It almost makes him look as if he knows something we don't know."

"Now that you mention it, Big Bill, Jabber does have that look," George said, smiling himself.

"But I want my smile to be bigger than Jabber's, if you don't mind, so there's absolutely no question of whether I'm smiling or not."

One day Big Bill's wife, Rosemary, called me just as I was leaving the office for lunch.

"Big Bill just fainted and put his head through the bottom panel of our front door, Doctor. Can you come right down or should I call an ambulance?"

"Is he conscious, Rosemary?"

"Oh yes, now he is. He's sitting on the floor holding a towel over his left eye where he has a big gash. He's swearing just like he did when he was a sergeant in the infantry in World War II."

"I'll be right over," I said.

Big Bill was still sitting on the floor and still swearing when I got there. He had a deep gash over his left eye.

"That's going to require suturing, Big Bill," I said. "It's down to the bone."

"Just a Band-Aid, that's all I need, Doctor. I don't want my fainting like this turned into a big event. Just bandage me up and I'll get on with my work."

"Do I ever tell you how to arrange flowers, Big Bill?" I said.

"No, no, I just don't want to be a bother to anybody."

I took him to the office and repaired his laceration. It required thirteen sutures. The whole area around his left eye was already black and blue. He would have a lot of explaining to do to all his friends, who knew his wife beat him up occasionally. I checked him over thoroughly. I found no abnormalities. His EKG was entirely normal.

"I just fainted, that's all, Doctor. It's no big fuss."

"Have you fainted like this before?" I said.

"Yes, as a matter of fact, I did. About a month ago. It happened while I was making a delivery. One of the flower arrangements flipped over when I took a corner. I stopped to fix it and I blacked out for a minute or two. It was nothing to worry about. When I came to, I completed the delivery and came back to the shop. I worked until eleven o'clock that night and didn't think anything of it."

"Did you have a warning that you were going to black out? Did you twitch or lose control of your bladder?"

"No, Doctor, nothing like that. If I had thought it was important, I would have called you. There was no warning and no twitching and I didn't wet my pants. It wasn't a seizure. Like I told you, it lasted about one minute and then I finished my delivery without any problems. It didn't bother me one bit."

I admitted Big Bill to the hospital even though he protested loudly. His skull x-rays were normal.

"I knew they would be," Big Bill said.

"So did I," I said. "It would take more than a one-inch door panel to crack that thick skull of yours, Big Bill."

I ordered a cardiac monitor.

"When am I getting out of here, Doctor? Remember, with me in the hospital, my wife has to do all the work herself, and she's an old lady, you know."

"You'd better not let her hear you say that, Big Bill, or I'll be stitching up your other eye," I said. "You'll get out in about three days if we find nothing."

"Exactly what are you looking for, Doctor?"

"You've had two unexplained fainting spells, so we know that something is going on even though we haven't been able to document it. What I suspect is a cardiac arrhythmia, a run of irregular beating or a period of asystole, which is a delay in the beat and the heart is completely still, causing you to black out. Your heart may actually skip several beats, causing your blood pressure to drop, and you faint. We call that syncope. Your own natural pacemaker in your heart that you were born with, is beginning to fail. We call that condition, "sick sinus syndrome."

"If I have that problem," Big Bill said, "what can be done about it?"

"We insert an artificial pacemaker and that will prevent any further attacks. It's a simple procedure and your problem is solved."

All the studies were negative. The cardiac monitor did not pick up any abnormal rhythms or short periods of asystole.

Big Bill was getting restless.

"You see, I told you so," he said. "It was just a simple fainting spell, after all."

"I'll discharge you today, Bill, but I want you to come into the office next week, and we'll repeat the cardiac monitor for another twenty-four hours while you're up and about."

"Do you really think that's necessary?"

"Yes, I do, Bill. I still think that you have a sick sinus syndrome."

"Well, why don't you just have a pacemaker inserted and I'll be on my way?"

"It's not that easy. Medicare requires documentation. You see, the bureaucrats no longer trust physicians so they will not accept our opinion without proper documentation."

"I've got enough money. Why don't we just forget about Medicare and I'll pay for it myself?"

"The pacemaker, alone, costs thousands of dollars. And doing it outside of Medicare is illegal. The law specifically forbids circumventing Medicare."

"I didn't know that," Big Bill said. "You mean to tell me that if I was a millionaire, I would still have to use Medicare?"

"If you enroll, there is no way you can get around it," I said.

"And I thought this was a free country," Bill said. "I guess the only truly free people in this country are the politicians in Congress."

"That's the law, unfortunately," I said.

"By the way, Doctor," Big Bill said, "Dr. Parker saw me in the hallway this morning. He's the urologist who put that stent in my right ureter last year to keep it open, remember? He told me as long as I'm already in the hospital, he would like to adjust and reposition the stent. He said it would only take about twenty minutes of general anesthesia and it would save me another trip to the hospital. I was scheduled to see him next week. All we need is your OK.''

"Bill, I would prefer to solve your present problem first before we subject you to a procedure that requires general anesthesia, even briefly.''

"I certainly don't want to come back to have that done, Doctor. Dr. Parker assured me that it's just a simple procedure and involves practically no risk at all. You haven't found anything specific on me during this hospitalization and he says there's really no contraindication.''

"Bill, you can go ahead with this procedure if you insist, but you'll have to have it done without my permission. The nurse will give you the necessary papers to sign.''

"By God, you're stubborn, Doctor!'' Big Bill said.

"It's your life, Bill. If you were my brother or father, I'd be just as stubborn.''

Dr. Parker scheduled the short procedure for the next morning, promising Bill that he would be discharged that same afternoon.

The procedure went along smoothly and was completed in twenty minutes, just as Dr. Parker had estimated. As Bill was ready to be moved to a stretcher to be taken to the recovery room, he developed a ventricular tachycardia that progressed rapidly to ventricular fibrillation. Repeated shocks to his heart failed to reverse this deadly arrhythmia. The resuscitation team worked on him for sixty minutes before they gave up and pronounced him dead.

At Big Bill's funeral, there were hundreds of people. It was one of the biggest funerals ever held in town. All the people in town loved this big guy and they were truly sorry to see him go.

They all commented how good Big Bill looked. They especially admired his big smile. It was not just a mystifying Mona Lisa smile.

"That's just the way he looked,'' somebody said, "the day he won the lottery. You can't look any better than that.''

Lessons To Be Learned

The cardiac muscle is a unique muscle that has the ability to contract rhythmically. This beating is initiated in the heart's own pacemaker called the sinoatrial node, as was mentioned in a previous chapter. This is a special bundle of cardiac fibers about 1.5 centimeters in length and is located in the lateral border of the right atrium at the junction of the superior vena cava, which is the large vein that drains blood from the head, neck, chest and upper arms.

The cells of the sinoatrial node initiate the spontaneous rhythmical beating of the heart by their capability of depolarization, which in turn stimulates adjacent cells. This electrical activity is then transmitted along special conducting cells to another node called the AV node (atrioventricular node) which lies beneath the right atrial endocardium. The depolarization is then transmitted along other specialized bundles of fibers, called the His-Purkinje network throughout the left and right sides of the heart. The electrical activity that develops in these specialized nodes and conducting fibers is what is recorded on the EKG and allows the physician to determine abnormalities such as arrhythmias and myocardial infarctions.

The sinoatrial node is rhythmical and controls the AV node in this aspect. However, there is a fail-safe mechanism in this system which allows the AV node to initiate the beat if the SA node is blocked or becomes inactive by disease or degeneration. In this case, however, the rhythm is irregularly irregular.

There is no doubt that we were dealing with brief episodes of a deadly cardiac arrhythmia in Big Bill's case that caused asystole, syncope, and then collapse. These episodes may appear relatively innocuous to the patient. Unfortunately for Bill, we were never able to document our impressions, which is not uncommon. The present restrictions by Medicare regarding the implantation of pacemakers and defibrillators have resulted in many unnecessary deaths. Of course, the other side of the coin is that many of the pacemakers in the past were implanted without the required specific criteria for implantation. Kickbacks from pacemaker manufacturers to surgeons were also discovered. So this led to the present restrictions. Abuse leads to restrictions which in turn lead to rationed care and this situation will only get worse as technology continues to explode.

The repositioning of the stent, of course, should have been delayed until we had settled the problem of Big Bill's arrhythmia. But he was in a hurry to get back to work. Unfortunately, after so much doctor bashing that has taken place in the newspapers and on TV news broadcasts, many patients feel that deeper investigation of a problem is only another method a physician uses to fatten his own purse. So the doctor finds himself surrendering to a patient's demands, hoping there will still be enough time in the future to document a definitive diagnosis. Unfortunately, as in this case, the next attack can end up being the last attack, and the doctor is left with the sad thought "if only I had continued to argue and persuade."

Chapter Twenty-eight

A Private Matter

*R*hoda St. John wouldn't be caught dead without a flask of Father John's Cough Elixir in her purse. She bought it by the quart, and every morning the first thing she did on arising was refill her silver flask and take a snort.

"It's not the alcohol, you know, Doctor, that is the beneficial constituent," she said during one of her visits. "The alcohol just facilitates the absorption of Father John's secret ingredient into the blood stream, but, of course, you know that already."

She'd smile and fondle her silver flask lovingly.

She used it for her arthritis, dyspepsia, headaches, lumbago, constipation, diarrhea, weakness, loss of appetite, insomnia, dizziness, deafness, sciatica, dandruff, and a million other ailments that plagued her over the years. Primarily, however, she used it for her cough. The fact that nobody had ever heard her cough for the last fifty years never bothered her at all.

Her daughter got very upset with her the Sunday before she fractured her hip. They were sitting in the front pew at the Our Lady of Mercy Church on Broad Street, where everybody could see them. Rhoda slipped out her silver flask during the eight o'clock service, and tilting her head farther back than she usually does, took an extra long swig, smacking her lips loudly as she recapped the flask. Her daughter jabbed her mother in the ribs with her elbow and whispered, *"Mother! Not in church!"*

Rhoda turned to her daughter slowly, like the Queen Mother turning to a misbehaving child, and said haughtily, "Do you want me to cough right in the middle of the service?"

"Nobody's heard you cough in this town for the last fifty years," her daughter whispered.

Rhoda held the silver flask up high in her right hand. It caught the light streaming through the stained-glass window with a brilliant reflection.

"I owe my good health to Father John," Rhoda declared, loud enough for the entire congregation to hear.

That was the last time they ever sat in the front pew.

One week later, Rhoda slipped on the steps to the church and fractured her right hip. When the ambulance came, she was sitting at the bottom of the stairs, her silver flask held tightly in her right hand. She had taken two swigs to ward off the devil and settle her stomach.

"Now careful, boys," she said to the ambulance attendants as they lifted her one-hundred-twenty-pound body into the ambulance. "You're transporting a delicate old lady here with exceptionally creaky old bones."

She had her hip pinned the next day and her post-operative course was essentially uneventful.

"I knew you'd do well, Rhoda," I said. "I was rooting for you."

She gave me a devilish look.

"I guess that makes you a 'Rhoda Rooter,' Doctor," she said smiling.

"How many snorts have you taken out of that magic flask of yours, Rhoda?" I said.

"Only two, Doctor, I swear to God," she said, holding up her right hand.

Her lab work indicated a moderate anemia, so I ordered the necessary blood studies, including a bone marrow.

The day after the hematologist had performed the bone marrow procedure, I walked into her room in the hospital at six in the morning. She was just waking up.

"Have you had your bone marrow test done, Rhoda?"

I spoke fairly loudly because she was moderately deaf, especially when she wanted to be.

"My bow and arrow test, Doctor?" she answered. "Yes, yes, I

did."

With that comment she reached for her flask and took a good swallow, as if to say, "Boy, I deserve some kind of compensation after they stuck that arrow into my poor old body."

Examination of the bone marrow revealed that she had pernicious anemia, a condition caused by the reduced ability of the body to absorb vitamin B12 from the gastrointestinal tract.

She had no trouble learning how to give herself B12 injections once a month.

"That is probably the only form of anemia that doesn't respond to Father John's Cough Elixir," she told me.

She did well with her physiotherapy program, and within three months she was back on her feet without a cane.

"Not bad for an eighty-year-old woman," she said, smiling at me. "But I couldn't have done it without the help of Father John."

With that statement, she took a hefty snort and smacked her lips, as if applying a period to the sentence she had just uttered.

I persuaded her to continue using her cane, even though she grumbled about it. She came to the office every three months to have her blood checked and to make sure she was taking her injections. It is so common for elderly patients to forget to take their medications. She gradually stretched her visits to six months. She would have gone to a yearly schedule but I objected because that would have been too long for a woman her age.

She had no further problems until, at the age of ninety-five, she slipped on the church steps again in exactly the same spot where she had fallen before. This time she shattered the left hip. She took three snorts out of her magic flask and sat there waiting for the ambulance, while her daughter stood beside her wringing her handkerchief.

I saw her in the emergency room of the hospital and ordered the necessary x-rays of her hip. She refused any medication for pain. Later, in her room, she asked me how bad the fracture was.

"Much worse than the first time, Rhoda," I said. "This time I believe the orthopedic surgeon will do a hip replacement and your actual rehabilitation, surprisingly, will be shorter than the first time."

"This time, Doctor, we will do it my way," she said.

"And what way is that, Rhoda?" I said, sitting on the edge of the bed, holding her right hand.

"You aren't going to get around me, Doctor, by holding my hand," she said. "I've made up my mind."

"Well, tell me, Rhoda, exactly what your plans are. I promise you that I'll do everything in my power to follow your wishes, within reason, and make you as comfortable as possible. After all, we both want you to get out of the hospital as soon as possible."

She looked at me directly, her blue eyes sharp and clear. There was no doubt that she had something on her mind and wasn't going to let anybody stand in her way.

"All I want is a moderate supply of Father John's Elixir and nothing more. I don't want any food and I don't want any B12 shots. And you have to promise me that you won't give me any intravenous fluids. Do you think you can arrange that without some inquisitive old judge sticking his nose into my business?"

"Have you spoken to your daughter and your sons about your decision, Rhoda?"

"Yes, I have, many times. They said they would accept my decision if you would allow it, even though they would hate to see me die before my rightful time. I told them that this is my rightful time. I have decided myself when to make my exit and there is no better moment than the present. By the time an individual is ninety-five and still has her wits about her, she should be allowed to say farewell when she thinks it's proper. Don't you agree, Doctor?"

"Yes, I do, Rhoda," I said, "but you must realize one thing, that when you depart from this world, your family and your friends and I are the ones left behind weeping."

She placed her hand on top of mine.

"Thank you, Doctor, you're very sweet," she said. "Now go to the nurses' station and leave the proper orders so that I won't be bothered."

She spoke to me like a mother would to her son.

I called her daughter. The entire family had already discussed their mother's plans. All of them were willing to allow Rhoda to have her last wish.

I wrote the necessary orders. The food trays were to be placed at her bedside and she could eat if she so desired.

All she took was an occasional swallow from her silver flask. She died in five days. No judges, lawyers, or governmental commissions were notified of her plans. Nobody attempted to interfere with her decision.

After all, this was a private matter.

LESSONS TO BE LEARNED

This was a simple case of an elderly lady, at ninety-five, who decided that enough was enough. Her only joy in life was drinking Father John's Cough Elixir. She had surgery and prolonged rehabilitation facing her after her second hip fracture.

She decided to take a different route. I suppose if one of the nurses had complained that we were committing murder by allowing the patient to make this decision, an interventionist judge might have caused a considerable amount of trouble. But the patient was ninety-five years old and everybody seemed to agree with her right of self-determination.

The family and I could have been dragged into the middle of a prolonged legal mess by our action. There are many prosecuting attorneys hanging around waiting to sink their teeth into a juicy opportunity like this to gain their 15 minutes of glory that Andy Warhol mentioned in his writings.

There is no doubt that self-determination is coming. It can't be stopped. And oddly, it won't be a moral issue. It will develop on economic grounds. And not even the U.S. Supreme Court nor any religious group will be able to stop it.

Chapter Twenty-nine

Out, Out, Damned Lumps

Jan Panek was an old Polish farmer. You didn't have to ask what he did for a living. Your nose told you. He raised chickens. He had one of the largest chicken farms in central Connecticut. He made a considerable amount of money raising and selling chickens. But it wasn't the thought of making money that made Jan Panek get up at the ungodly hour of four o'clock in the morning and work until ten at night. He simply loved to work. As far as he was concerned, there was nothing else to do in this world except raise chickens. Everybody called him the Polish Chicken Man. While he worked, he kept up a constant chatter in Polish. The chickens were Rhode Island Reds, but to Jan, they were Polish Reds.

"Ah, moje malutkie kochane czerwonie ptaszki, Witam was wszystkie dzis rano."

("Ah, my little beloved red birds, good morning to you all.")

And the clucking chorus he received as he entered the hen houses was a joy to his heart.

There was no room in his life for doctors. The only "medicine" he took was two ounces of Polish vodka every night before he went to bed.

About one month before he came to see me, a general weariness overcame him. It became difficult for him to get out of bed in the morning. Instead of getting up at four as he usually did, it would be five or even six before he started his daily chores. He began to take naps in the afternoon. He attributed these symptoms to old age. After all, he said to himself, I am seventy years old, time, maybe, to say good-by to my feathery friends. One night, as he was taking a bath, he noticed a lump under the skin of his abdomen. It was painless, hard, and immovable. What am I growing here, an egg? After all these years raising chickens, am I turning into a chicken? He began to worry and it wasn't like him to waste time worrying. Every night, from then on, he would palpate the lump. My egg is growing, he would say to himself. It would be wise to make arrangements for my departure.

A second lump soon appeared on the right side of his chest. Every night after his bath, he carried on a debate with himself. Should I see the doctor? My chicken body is producing more eggs. The doctors will take one look and they will immediately want to operate. That surely would be the end. That happened to one of his friends. Expose the cancer to air and you are gone in a flash, he thought. When death is knocking on your door, that is no time to go visit the doctor. You just have to work harder and faster to stay one step ahead of the "widmo smiertelny" (grim reaper). Perhaps he would be lucky and drop dead as he tended his "kochane ptaszki" (beloved birds). Or better yet, perhaps he would die in his sleep.

So he waited and continued the debate for three months. By that time he had a total of eight hard, immovable lumps scattered over his chest, back and abdomen. The increasing fatigue finally forced him to come into my office.

"I dead man, Pan Doktor," he said sadly.

"Why do you say that, Jan?" I said.

"Because I have lumps like eggs from my chickens all over chest and belly. Three months now and I get very tired. Pretty soon, I think I go to sleep forever."

"Let me see your lumps, Jan," I said.

He stripped to the waist.

"Zapodziewac przeklete guzy" ("Out, out, damned lumps"), he said, pointing to the largest one below his umbilicus.

I checked him over completely and found nothing except the lumps. He was a wiry old man with no fat on his work-hardened body. I drew blood for a battery of screening tests, hoping I could find a clue. A chest x-ray was negative.

"What you think, Pan Doktor?" Jan said. "I finished, yes?"

"Jan," I said, "you do have a serious problem, but it's too early to say you're finished. Your physical examination, except for the lumps, is entirely negative. I believe you do have a cancer somewhere in your body and these lumps are the sign that it's spreading."

"So I dead man." Jan said.

"No, you're not," I said. "There are a few things we have to do first, to see if you have a cancer that can be treated."

"What you want to do, Pan Doktor?" Jan said.

"I'd like to put you in the hospital for a few days, do some more x-rays, and then take out one of those lumps. When we examine it under the microscope, we can find out what part of your body it came from. Then we can decide if it can be treated."

"No hospital," Jan said, waving his right hand in disgust. "No more blood. I go back to chicken farm and work till die."

We discussed the problem for over an hour. Jan was stubborn, but I persisted and finally he relented. He agreed to the excision of the largest lump as an outpatient if I promised that he could go right back to work as soon as it was done.

I made the necessary arrangements with the hospital and a general surgeon. The procedure was done under local anesthesia. I stood by Jan's side and watched. He muttered "goddamn" only once during the thirty minutes it took to remove his malignant "egg."

Unfortunately, the microscopic examination of the mass gave us no clue as to its origin. It was a highly anaplastic cancer that resembled no specific tissue in the body.

He came back to my office one week later to have his sutures removed.

"I no like meat cutter in hospital," he said. "Pan Doktor, you take stitches out, please."

I assured him the surgeon was a highly skilled and well-liked individual, but Jan wasn't listening to me.

"What you find, Pan Doktor?" he said, eager to get some answers.

"I'm sorry to say, Jan, that the lump did not reveal its origin. All I can say is that it's a cancer. Where it came from, we simply don't know."

"Hah!" Jan said. "I know now I should stay home and take care of chickens. Dowidzenia, Pan Doktor. Good-bye."

"Wait a minute, Jan," I said. "I'll give you another appointment. I want to see you in two weeks."

"No, no, no," Jan said. "For why?"

"To watch you and make sure you don't have any pain," I said. "I want you to be as comfortable as possible."

"I go home now and die," Jan said. "If I need you, Pan Doktor, I come to see you."

I gave him a return appointment for one month even though he made a disagreeable face when I handed him the card. I knew he would eventually need me as the cancer gradually overwhelmed his body.

"If you don't come to my office, Jan, I will come to your chicken farm," I said. "There is no way you can escape from me."

I put my arm around his shoulders.

"You understand, Jan?"

"I understand, Pan Doktor."

I really didn't expect him to show up for his appointment the following month. But the day of his appointment, I detected the unmistakable odor of chickens in the hallway of my office.

"Jan is here?" I said to the nurse, pleasantly surprised.

"Room three, Pan Doktor," she said smiling.

Jan looked much better. He had obviously gained some weight, five pounds according to the nurse's notes.

"Do you feel better, Jan?" I said.

"Yes, Pan Doktor," he said. "I much better. And lumps, they start to go."

The lumps were about half the size they had been originally. They also felt much softer.

"Yes, Jan," I said as I checked each one. "They are definitely going away."

"Why they go away, Pan Doktor?" Jan said.

"I don't know why, Jan," I said. "You understand our immune system?"

"No," Jan said.

"When you were a child, Jan, you got a smallpox vaccination on your left arm," I said. "You see the scar here. That prevented you from getting smallpox."

"Yes, I understand smallpox, Pan Doktor," Jan said.

"Well, when you had your operation to remove that big lump, that was just like a smallpox vaccination. Apparently, it started to make you immune to the cancer, and the lumps are now melting away."

"I understand," Jan said.

"The answer to your malignant tumors is right here in your body, Jan," I said. "And I wish we knew what that answer is. Unfortunately, we don't have many people like you whose bodies are curing their cancers. If we knew the answer, we could save thousands of lives."

Jan indicated he didn't give a damn about the thousands of people we could save. He just wanted to get back to his chickens.

"Dowidzenia, Pan Doktor," Jan said. "Good-bye."

"I shall see you in one month, Jan," I said.

This time he didn't give me an argument.

Over a period of three months, all his lumps disappeared except one, and that was one-quarter its original size. The following three months, that last lump remained the same. I again persuaded Jan to have that one excised. It took about an hour of arguing to overcome his objections. I was counting on the surgery to give his immune system another jolt.

He had the final lump excised the next day. I knew that waiting several days could have caused him to change his mind. The path report was identical to the first lump, a highly anaplastic carcinoma of undetermined origin.

One week later, Jan was in the office for removal of his sutures.

"That is bad thing when you make me have last lump cut out," he said. He looked very unhappy. "I have so much pain there now."

The incision was well healed with no evidence of inflammation. I tried to reassure him.

"I make big mistake, Pan Doktor," he said. "Dowidzenia. Good-by."

I saw him two more times, a month apart. He had no signs of recurrence and had regained all his old stamina. He got up at four in the morning without complaining and worked until ten at night. But he expressed considerable bitterness about the decision to excise the last lump.

"Why you make me do it, Pan Doktor?" he said on his last visit.

"Because I thought it was the best thing to do," I said.

He wagged his head.

"Bad, bad mistake," he said. "Much pain now."

He pulled out a bottle from a brown bag he had brought into the office. He handed it to me.

"This is best Polish vodka, Pan Doktor. Better than smallpox needle. Every night, you take two ounces before bed. You sleep like baby. I think maybe best medicine for lumps and everything else. Dowidzenia, Pan Doktor, good-bye. You make bad mistake last lump, but you still good doktor."

I never saw Jan again, but I checked with his nephew. The old stubborn mule was still going strong, now well into his eighties. I know that he is undoubtedly still complaining of pain in the site of the last lump that was removed from his wiry old body. I've heard from a variety of sources that vodka is good for that.

LESSONS TO BE LEARNED

We have here a stubborn old man who hated to go to the doctor. He lived in his own universe, his own "hen house," and didn't care a whit about anything else or anybody else.

Something triggered the immune system in his body when that first lump was excised. This released a multitude of killer cells that had the malignancy zeroed in as the target.

It is unfortunate that few medical centers are investigating this phenomenon. Patients like this old man should be given free care and other incentives and persuaded to allow themselves to be studied. The answers are right there. We have to work harder to find them.

We probably would have lost this patient if we hadn't spent the time in persuading him to have that first lump removed. That was obviously what triggered the immune response. Among the body's defenses in the blood stream are Helper T cells and Suppressor T cells. The immune response is enhanced by the former and blocked by the latter.

Recent studies indicate that such a minor thing as exposure to ultra violet B radiation (equivalent to 20 minutes of sunlight) releases Suppressor T cells, thereby causing the patient to be more vulnerable to various skin cancers. Individuals living in Florida have an incidence of skin cancer 15 times greater than those living in New England.

Studies also show that patients who undergo tonsillectomies have an incidence of leukemia eight times greater than individuals who retain those sentinels of the throat.

As time goes on, other factors that enhance or block the immune system will be discovered and medical care will change dramatically.

Chapter Thirty

Catching Rainbows

Governor John Harper Trumbull was obviously dying. His lips were blue and his face an ashen gray. He was gasping for air and every breath was an agonizing effort. His neck veins were bulging and his legs were swollen twice their normal size. He was drowning in his own body fluids and yet, there he was sitting in his favorite chair smoking a big fat cigar, coughing, snorting, and choking on a mixture of frothy mucus and smoke. His eyes glazed over frequently and his mind drifted in and out of reality.

He had been sent home from the hospital to die peacefully and quietly in his own familiar surroundings. But at the moment he didn't look very comfortable, peaceful, or quiet.

"I guess," he said haltingly and with some difficulty, "that the deadly tide...is finally...coming in." He managed a weak smile and took another puff on his cigar.

Florence Coolidge, his daughter, had called me the day before.

"Apparently, there is nothing much that can be done for my father. He seems to have lost the will to live. The doctors in Hartford have given up. They said that he can't last more than a few days or weeks at the most. So they discharged him and advised me to have a local physician care for him at home."

The Governor was suffering from end-stage intractable congestive heart failure. He was no longer responding to standard diuretic therapy.

It was 1961. His greatest moments had been in the far distant past when he served as governor of the State of Connecticut from 1925 to 1931. He had been a staunch Republican businessman, having founded the Trumbull Electric Manufacturing Company in Plainville in 1899, along with his brother Henry and a friend, Frank Wheeler. In 1908, he and the others organized the Plainville Trust Company. He was its president for forty-seven years.

The Governor had been a devoted aviator. He became known as the "Flying Governor" during his tenure in the Capitol in Hartford. He had many mishaps in the air and survived a number of serious crashes with his planes in the days before Charles Lindbergh made his epochal flight to Paris.

Knowing that he had been an ardent fisherman in his younger days, I stood directly in front of him on that first day I came to his house to examine him. I aroused him from his lethargy and said, "Do you want to go fishing for rainbow trout again?"

I could see that he was surprised by the question.

"In this condition?" he said, shaking his head. "You know that's impossible, Doctor. I'm at the end of my journey."

"Nothing is impossible, Governor," I said. "If you really want to go fishing again, you'll have to help me. I can't make you better all by myself."

"Are you going to restore my youth?" he said cynically.

"No," I said. "That's really impossible, and you know it. All I'm going to do is give you some extra time if you're willing to help. But if you'd rather sit there in a cloud of smoke and drown in your own body fluids like a rat trapped in an underground sewer, that's your decision."

"The doctors in the hospital weren't so optimistic," he said. "They sent me home to die."

"You do have a serious condition, Governor. I'm not going to minimize it. But it certainly isn't hopeless. If the doctors in Hartford gave you that impression, they're wrong. But if you're convinced that you're going to die and you've lost your will to live, then it will be very difficult to prevent you from dying. If you're half the fighter I suspect you are, you won't depart from this life without putting up a good battle. I want you to remember the great times you've had fishing all over this country. Don't lose sight of that vision. There's no reason why we can't get you back into shape to go fishing again. Are you ready to fight?

I put out my hand.

He hesitated a moment, but then responded.

"I am ready to do battle, Doctor," he said weakly.

I could see by the look on his face that he was not entirely convinced of his ability to win this last struggle.

After all, at eight-eight he was a very old man in dire straits, absolutely sure he was going to die, his brain numbed by illness and advanced age, confused by the incomprehensible fusion of the past and the present, his heart fluttering erratically and weakening with every passing moment. His atherosclerotic kidneys were unable to excrete the body fluids that were flooding the microscopic air sacs of his lungs, preventing oxygen from reaching his vital organs. He was, as he suspected, very close to death. Wasn't he sent home to do just that? Discussing fishing at this time was like teasing him with the impossible visions of heaven as he had lived it in his past years of glory.

"First, the cigar has to go," I said.

"Now, wait a minute, Doctor," he said. "If I'm going to die, it's going to be with a cigar in my mouth."

"Who's talking about dying?" I said. "I'm talking about going fishing. I'll be in charge temporarily until we have you back in shape. I want you to think, talk, and dream fishing. Just see yourself holding your favorite rod and suddenly feeling that quick jerk as the trout takes your fly."

"Remember," he said. "This is only a temporary arrangement. I'm still the boss."

"How can I forget," I said. "You keep reminding me. You know, you're a stubborn old mule."

"Yes," he said, "and an old bastard besides."

I started the Governor on a different diuretic that had just come on the market a few weeks before. I also decreased his digitalis medication because his racing pulse and the frequent premature contractions of his heart indicated he was overdigitalized. His kidneys were not able to excrete the digitalis normally and it was gradually building up in his body to an excess that eventually could trigger a lethal arrhythmia. By increasing his dose of sublingual nitroglycerin, his exertional angina virtually disappeared.

His response was dramatic. The edema in his legs subsided rapidly. I added potassium to his regimen because of the loss of this electrolyte in his edema fluid and in one week the Governor had lost about twenty pounds of fluid and could breathe fairly easily.

"This is, indeed, a miracle," he said, "and I can't think of a better way of celebrating this momentous occasion than by lighting up and puffing away."

His blood pressure was normal when he wasn't smoking. Ten minutes on a cigar and his blood pressure rose to 200/110 with a pulse of 110.

"We didn't travel down this road just to have you blow it all to hell with your cigars, Governor," I said.

"All right, all right," he said. "I'll cut it back to five minutes."

Within a month, I could see that he was about ready to go fishing. He had already informed me that he was a strict fly fisherman and gave me a look of utter contempt when I told him I like to fish with worms.

"I can't believe it" he said, clucking his tongue and blowing out a cloud of smoke that made me cough.

"I've never been successful fishing with flies in Connecticut, Governor," I said.

"Well, when we go to my private pond in Moodus, Doctor, I promise you'll catch plenty of trout with flies," he answered. "It's so heavily stocked that the fish have to swim shoulder to shoulder."

"I didn't know fish had shoulders," I said.

"See how much you have to learn, Doctor?" he said.

He laughed and slapped his thigh with the joy of anticipation. He nearly slipped out of his chair in the process.

"Do you have the necessary fly-fishing equipment, or would you like to use some of mine?" he asked.

"Well, at the moment, I have a seven and one-half foot Browning rod with medium action, tapered leaders at four pounds test, and a tapered floating-sinking line," I said. "Is that adequate?"

"Adequate, adequate," he said, grunting and blowing out more smoke and waving his right hand. "And how about flies?"

"I had my best luck years ago when I was still fly fishing at Natchaug State Forest and the Salmon River with a modified Red Ibis on a number six hook," I said.

"That sounds interesting," he said. "I favor a modified Silver Ghost or a Red Devil, myself. As for leaders, I am sure you know that ideally they should be invisible to the fish. Since that is relatively impossible, I use the finest tippet to allow the fly to land on the water and behave as naturally as the real thing. For trout you'll need a leader that is eight thousandths to six thousandths of an inch. And trout feeding on small insects require a fly no larger than the natural food they're taking. Landing a decent trout with a fine leader requires the sensitivity of a violin virtuoso to set the hook properly, not the violent action you usually see among the local fishermen on our streams and ponds."

Now the Governor was warming up to his favorite subject. The fog that usually clouded his brain had dissipated, and there was a new bright look in his eyes. A few more puffs on his cigar filled the room with smoke, causing him to squint and cough. He forgot all about his five-minute limit with the cigar.

"The rod, of course, is an extremely important part of the whole setup," he continued, not waiting for me to answer in any way. "All fishermen know that. One of the early rod makers in the nineteenth century was a man named Phillippe from Easton, Pennsylvania, a gunsmith and violin maker who fished and later designed the Stradivarius of fly rods. In 1870, three years before I was born, a man named Hiram Leonard began varnishing rods in Bangor, Maine. He was an expert who created a seven and one-half foot artistic achievement out of bamboo consisting of two pieces with an extra tip, each of which was made up of six separate but equal slices of bamboo. Subsequently, men like Thomas, Edwards, and the elder Payne learned the art of rod making from the old master himself.

"This is the kind of rod I prefer, a split bamboo with a light tip that gives you the sweet feel that is impossible to duplicate with other materials. Orvis makes a beautiful cane varnished to a warm dark brown that glows like a winter fire on a cold and nasty day. It is interesting to note that the shape of the cork grip frequently identifies the maker.

"But even more important is the reel. You need one with a drag that requires the same feeling as hitting the proper harmonic high on the E string of a violin. Fritz Kreisler would have made a fine fisherman, and for all I know, he probably did fish in Austria, where he was born.

"As for the fish, you need a certain cunning and ingenuity to catch rainbow trout. This is the most elegant of all freshwater fish, with the sparkling, flashing brilliance of his fiery sides as he turns with his powerful body and then fades from view as you see his olive-colored back disappearing among similarly colored rocks. Is he still there, you wonder, hiding under a projecting ledge, just as cunning himself, having learned to be wary of the fisherman who keeps waving his magic wand above the cold, clean, rushing waters of the magnificent rivers and brooks of this country?"

The Governor's eyes gradually dimmed, his chin sagged to his chest, and he began to snore gently, his brain exhausted by the memories that had come flooding back. I took the cigar that he still clenched in his fingers and put it in the ashtray.

It was a beautiful spot in Moodus and we were on the pond early in the morning on a bright sunny day. The Governor was right. The pond was heavily stocked with rainbow trout and the fish were swimming shoulder to shoulder.

The Governor had a guide to help him climb into a rowboat. And there he sat in the middle of the boat looking like the Prince of Wales, while the guide paddled to the center of the pond, attached a fly to his line and proceeded to cast until he had about thirty or forty feet of line out in a billowing U. He then handed the pole to the Governor as the fly settled delicately on the smooth surface of the water.

There was an immediate hit, a large rainbow trout striking like a marauding shark, whipping the water into a violent splash as the Governor set the hook. With a mighty lunge the fish cleared the surface, enveloped in a fine spray, then danced on its tail in a wild convulsion, the Governor playing him like a master, the line taut but responding quickly to repeated dives and thrusts into the air, the fish twisting and turning, flashing its beautiful colors in its mad, agonizing attempts to free itself.

Finally, with the fish totally exhausted and by the side of the boat, the Governor handed the rod to the guide, who quickly netted the fish and removed the hook.

Another quick cast and the scene was repeated. It was déjà vu.

By the time I had my first fly attached and ready for the cast, the Governor had brought in three fish.

I cast my line out upon the still surface of the pond expecting an immediate strike like the Governor's first cast. Nothing happened, so I gave the fly an enticing twitch or two that would have driven any normal trout absolutely wild. Again nothing happened.

As I gradually pulled the line in, making the fly dance in erratic gyrations, I saw a twenty-inch rainbow follow it right up to the boat then turn up its nose.

"Why, you ____," I muttered between clenched teeth.

I cast the line again and again with the same result, all the fish pulsing their gills contemptuously in the clear, calm water and smirking as they turned away.

By noon I had tried at least thirty different flies with no success. And all the while the Governor was hauling in the fish as though he had a net on the end of his line instead of a fly. Red Devil, Silver Ghost, Black Gnat, Red Ibis, and all the others I had brought. I tried them all. Nothing worked.

We broke for lunch, the Governor chuckling all the way to the clubhouse.

"I think they know you're a worm fisherman, and so they're not biting deliberately," he laughed again as we leisurely went through a tuna fish salad and coffee.

"I've never seen so many fish with contemptuous smirks on their faces," I said. "They're actually behaving as though they represent a superior form of life. Don't they realize they are mere fish and they've been put on the earth to please man?"

"Are you talking about fish or women?" the Governor asked, still chuckling.

The afternoon was a repetition of the morning's fiasco. I didn't get one single strike while the Governor was hauling in rainbows until I thought his boat would sink from the sheer weight of the fish.

By the end of the day, he had more than two dozen fish and I didn't have one. However, he was gracious enough not to ridicule my fishing abilities.

"Don't worry," he said. "You'll get the hang of it sooner or later. After all, I've been fly fishing for a good many years."

On the way home, I could see the Governor was very pleased

with himself. As we drove up a long hill in Middletown, we approached a cemetery.

"Turn left there," he said. "I'm not ready for that place yet."

He looked and acted as if he had a new lease on life. He had no angina, no shortness of breath, and his brain was functioning remarkably well.

Back home he split the rainbow trout with me.

"Let's do this again in two weeks, Doctor," he said.

"That will be great, Governor," I said. "By then, I'll have a whole new set of flies to try out. And next time, I am also taking along a baseball bat so I can club them into submission if I don't catch any. I'll teach them not to smirk at me and turn up their noses in that insufferably superior manner they have."

I could still hear him laughing as I pulled out of the driveway.

Two weeks later, we were back at the pond in Moodus. The day was overcast and chilly that early in the morning, but absolutely perfect for fishing. The same guide was there, checking the temperature of the water.

"Ideal," he said, as he stood up and put the thermometer back into its case. "Fifty degrees."

He helped the Governor into the boat and then looked back at me.

"I'm sure you'll have better luck today," he said, shoving off and climbing into the boat.

By the time I was ready to cast, the Governor had already hooked two beauties.

I tried every trick known to mankind, but again was totally unsuccessful with the new batch of flies I had bought. By noon, I was ready to pummel the fish to death with the oars, but thought the Governor would look upon this method as unsportsmanlike. How much frustration can one man tolerate, I thought to myself.

About noon, the Governor broke for lunch, so I rowed over to the shore where he was slowly getting out of his boat.

"If you don't mind, Governor, I'd like to fish right through lunch. I promise you I'll have some trout in this boat by the time you get back, even if I have to jump in and grab them with my bare hands."

The Governor turned up the hill laughing. The guide, in the meantime, secured the boat on the shore and as he passed, threw me a blue coffee can.

"Here, try these special flies," he said. "The Governor doesn't know it, but these damn fish won't take a regular fly."

He winked at me and hurried up the hill behind the Governor. I opened the can and saw a glorious tangle of the juiciest looking night crawlers I had ever seen in my entire life. Aha, I thought to myself. Here is, no doubt, the secret to successful trout fishing. With the Governor's cataracts preventing close scrutiny, he hadn't noticed that the guide used worms to get a strike.

I wasted no time putting a worm on a hook and casting the line out about thirty feet. I was standing up in the boat at the time of the strike and it was an utterly magnificent thing to see. The fish broke the surface of the water with a powerful thrust, twisting and turning as he sliced through the air in an agony of motion, the spray catching the light in a dazzling iridescent swirl as he tail-danced for a good six feet. He then dove under the boat and in a desperate attempt to maintain the tautness of the line, I stepped back and hit the seat of the boat with the back of my leg, losing my balance and landing headfirst in the water. Now it was man against fish, and all my primitive instincts pumped adrenaline into my already racing blood. I kept the line taut throughout the fall, spitting water out of my mouth in a fine jet and yelling with exhilaration.

"Go ahead and turn up your nose and smirk, you writhing devil," I yelled out.

For a moment, I was Ahab and that trout was the great white whale.

The rainbow dove in a series of intricate maneuvers, first down deep, then under the boat and back, and finally into the air again before suddenly tiring. I brought him close to the boat and gently lifted him into the air.

He was a magnificent looking specimen, much too beautiful to allow him to die. I removed the hook and carefully put him back into the water. With three or four flips of his tail he was gone, but I could have sworn that when he was about ten feet away he turned around to look at me. There was no smirk on his face, just a look of genuine respect.

By the time the Governor came back, I had caught and released about ten beautiful rainbow trout, the smallest of the lot being eighteen inches. It was as if the word had gone out that I was a worthy opponent and the fish had decided to be cooperative.

During the rest of the afternoon, I caught six more fish using flies, proving the point that the fish had changed their attitude towards me. I held up each one for the governor to see and I heard the guide describing the fish as I gently let it go.

"I knew you'd catch on, Doctor," the Governor yelled out.

He was happy that I had finally caught some trout and I was pleased with the day's fishing, even though I kept remembering Samuel Johnson's definition of a fishing pole: "A stick with a fish on one end and a fool on the other."

As we drove home, I looked at the Governor sitting next to me. He hadn't even noticed that I was soaking wet. He was smiling to himself, very happy with the world.

"You know, Governor," I said, "you have a very good guide down there in Moodus."

"I know that, Doctor," he said. He was silent for a while. "Actually, I have two good guides."

"Two?" I said.

"Yes. One that helps me fish and one that gives me a little more time on this glorious planet."

He continued to smile. I knew he felt good.

I felt good, too.

About one week later, while examining the Governor, I found a small basal cell carcinoma on his left cheek.

"It's a superficial lesion, Governor," I explained to him. "It can be taken off easily under local anesthesia in the office using a skin curette followed by electrodesiccation."

"No," the Governor said. "If I have a cancer on my cheek, I'll have it cut out by a surgeon in the hospital the right way, under general anesthesia."

"First of all, Governor," I said, "you cannot tolerate general anesthesia. And secondly, this type of lesion does not warrant the added hazard of being put to sleep. Curettage under local anesthesia followed by electrodesiccation will give you the same result as surgical excision without the increased risk. Either method results in a three to four per cent recurrence rate. And if it does recur, it's a simple procedure to remove it again using the same dermatological method."

"I've made up my mind, Doctor, and you cannot change it. I shall have this cancer removed surgically under general anesthesia in the hospital and that's final."

The Governor made his own arrangements for the surgery to take place the following week. He did not go fishing for rainbows again. He died on May 21, 1961, and was buried three days later in Plainville, Connecticut.

LESSONS TO BE LEARNED

Frequently, a physician will see, if he is astute enough, treatment that will fail in the hospital but be successful at home. A slight change here and there in the treatment program, a more humanistic approach to the patient, an awakening of the patient to what interests him, and what unfolds before our eyes can appear to be as startling as a miracle.

Here was a man who was bed-ridden, suffering from intractable congestive heart failure, failing rapidly in the hospital, and by going home and being given a reason to live, suddenly turned the corner and started to improve.

But the very individuals and the institution that doomed him in the first place, still managed to lead him quickly to the grave when a minor procedure was done under general anesthesia.

Patients forget that general anesthesia is a rigidly controlled poisoning of the body, allowing surgery to be performed painlessly. But one should never forget that even though the death rate from anesthesia is relatively low, death still occurs. The elderly, already debilitated by disease and advanced age, are not the only ones who succumb. The young and healthy individuals undergoing simple surgical procedures are also its victims. And in many cases, we don't even understand why.

There's no doubt I surrendered to the Governor too soon. I tried to argue, but looking back, it appears to me to have been a feeble attempt to dissuade the Governor. I should have been more forceful. I didn't believe the city physicians would actually use general anesthesia for such a simple task. But just as I bent under the Governor's decision, apparently they did, too. And so, we've had to live with the memory of that event. What happened to the Governor, however, was

PATIENT BEWARE—

like a trigger in my brain that forced me not to surrender in similar encounters with other patients that occurred subsequently.

Chapter Thirty-one

The Twenty-Five Percent Protocol

"*T*he resident physician at the University Medical Center is on the phone, Doctor," the nurse said.

"Good," I said. "He's probably calling about Charlie Stoughton, the patient I sent there last week."

It *was* the resident.

"Doctor, I'm calling you about Mr. Stoughton. We'd like to start him on the Interferon Protocol, but he refuses to do so until we speak to you and get your OK."

He sounded irritated.

"Yes," I said. "I spoke to Mr. Stoughton just last night. He told me what you had planned for him. Has Dr. Prouter seen him?"

I had sent Charlie Stoughton to Dr. Prouter for admission and work-up. I knew that many times the residents took charge of referred patients in the University Center Hospital with very little supervision from the staff physicians.

"I'm calling for Dr. Prouter," the resident said, slightly more irritated.

"Why do you want to put him on the Interferon Protocol?" I said.

"He's next on the list and we don't have enough patients treated with Interferon yet to make the statistics valid. You did send him to be treated here, didn't you, Doctor?"

"Yes, I did. I sent him to Dr. Prouter for conventional therapy for his lymphocytic lymphoma. What is the remission rate for the Interferon Protocol?"

I already knew the answer. The Swedes had reported a twenty-five percent remission rate over six months ago.

"Twenty-five percent," the resident said. He sounded huffy.

In presentations of cases by residents at the medical school, local doctors are referred to as "LMDs," usually in moderately derisive tones. It carries over from the disdain the resident staff develops from cases that have been mishandled on the outside and then referred to the University Medical Center for treatment.

"And what is the remission rate with conventional therapy?" I said.

"Well...it approaches one hundred percent, as you probably already know," he said.

"Then why do you want to start him on the Interferon Protocol when I sent him there purposely for conventional therapy, Doctor?"

This time I added a slight edge to my voice.

"We have a grant to investigate the efficacy of the Interferon Protocol, Doctor," he said, his voice less irritated.

"Would you place your brother on the Interferon Protocol if he presented himself there for treatment, Doctor?" I said.

"No, of course not," the resident said. "That's an entirely different matter."

"*Is it now?*" I said. "When I send my patients to the University Medical Center, I don't want them placed on a protocol that has already been proved by the Swedes over six months ago to be inferior to conventional therapy. I consider my patients to be extensions of my own body. They are members of my family. When you finally end up in private practice, I hope you'll do the same. I would not accept a treatment protocol for one of my patients that I wouldn't accept for myself. Do you think that's unreasonable, Doctor?"

"Yes, I do," he said. "My task with this grant is to repeat the same protocol used by the Swedes to see if their results are valid. How are we going to accomplish that if all physicians felt like you?"

"Doctor," I said, "you will have to get your patients elsewhere, but *not* from me."

Charlie Stoughton had come into the office two weeks before. He wasn't his usual wise-cracking self and he didn't have any new jokes to tell me, so I knew he was worried about something. I had been treating him for diabetes for the last ten years. He had initially controlled his blood sugar with diet alone. After several years, I had to add an oral medication to his program to keep the blood sugar at a reasonable level. This held him for five years, but he finally progressed to insulin. On this last visit, however, he had two lumps just below his right inguinal ligament in his groin.

"I think I've got a hernia," he said.

"No, Charlie," I said, after the examination. "Those lumps are lymph nodes. Are they tender?"

"No," he said. "They just suddenly popped up from nowhere."

"These lymph nodes, or glands, as most people call them, are small filtering stations in our system of lymphatics. Our lymphatic system is similar to our vascular system of arteries and veins, but not as clearly defined. There is a constant flow of lymph, which is a faintly pale, yellow liquid, through these channels in between the various tissues of our body. It flows up to our neck where it finally empties into our veins. If the lymph nodes were infected, they would be tender to touch. But other diseases can affect these nodes. To make a proper diagnosis in many cases, we have to excise the nodes and examine them under the microscope."

Charlie agreed to have the nodes excised as an out-patient. He had two separate clusters adjacent to each other, the upper one being larger. Even though I had asked the surgeon to excise both clusters, he removed only the smaller, lower bunch. The path report described these as normal. Charlie was definitely upset when he found out he had to go through a second surgical procedure to remove the larger cluster of nodes. This time the pathologist reported what I had suspected: lymphocytic lymphoma. This is a malignant disorder of the lymph nodes.

I discussed the diagnosis with Charlie and his family. They decided to have him treated at the University Medical Center. I made the necessary arrangements and a week after his admission there, I received the call from the resident regarding the Interferon Protocol.

After my discussion with the resident, I received no further follow-up until three weeks later when Charlie's daughter called me.

"My father is dying," she said.

"I haven't received any information regarding your father since I refused to let them proceed with that treatment program that I felt wasn't right for him," I said.

"He has become very anemic and he's getting a unit of blood every three days," she said. "He's very depressed and cries all the time. Everybody's upset. We discussed this with the whole family. My father wants to die at home and we feel that's where he belongs."

I called Charlie's physician at the University Medical Center. He was very unhappy with the family's decision.

"We're not even half-way through our treatment," he said.

Charlie was discharged the next day, after signing the necessary forms absolving the hospital and all the physicians of any responsibility. I saw him at home the same day.

"How do I look?" he said.

"You look awful," I said.

"I want a second opinion," he said, managing a weak smile. We had played this routine before, when he hadn't been so deathly ill.

"All right, you're ugly, too," I said.

This time he laughed out loud.

"God, it's good to be home," he said. "I missed hearing all these wonderful compliments."

Charlie's hemoglobin was 8.0 grams. A normal reading is 14.5-15.5 grams. His diabetes was under good control on twenty units of NPH insulin. I added iron to his program. We all expected him to die. In two weeks his hemoglobin rose to 10.0 grams and he gained three pounds. Two weeks later it was 12. Six weeks after his discharge from the hospital, his hemoglobin leveled off at 13.5, and he had gained a total of six pounds.

Charlie was like his old self again, telling me a new joke with every visit. I matched joke for joke. He had received a total of six units of packed red cells while he was in the hospital. After his discharge, he had received no blood and had been maintained on iron alone, along with his insulin.

"If I hadn't been discharged from that hospital," he said a short time later, "I would have been dead in another two weeks. I don't know what they were giving me, but it sure was deadly."

I called the University Medical Center several times for the hospital summaries but I never received any. Charlie continued to do well without any specific treatment for his lymphocytic lymphoma.

His decision to die at home actually saved his life. He finally died of a heart attack at the age of seventy-eight, ten years after his discharge from the University Medical Center Hospital.

LESSONS TO BE LEARNED

There are patients with lymphocytic lymphoma on record that have normal life spans without any specific treatment. Charlie Stoughton was one of these patients. Whatever he was receiving in the hospital was killing him by destroying his bone marrow, the site of his red blood cell formation. He required a transfusion of one unit of red blood cells every 3 days while in the hospital. After his discharge, he received nothing but oral iron. There's no doubt that whatever treatment he was receiving was deadly. The hospital even withheld the records, which I'm sure, were damning. He may have been placed on the interferon or some other protocol after all.

The truth was Charlie's lymphoma was not progressive. It suddenly popped out in his right groin and was then clinically dormant. He required no treatment. This is the type of case that can distort statistics because no matter what the treatment consists of, if the patient survives, the treatment will get the credit; and if the patient dies, the disease gets the blame.

The problem for physicians is the difficulty in choosing a protocol that consists of watchful waiting and careful observation. As revealed in previous chapters, this too can end up in disaster. Unbearable pressure can be applied on the physician by the patient and the family. "Why isn't the doctor doing something" is a cry too often heard in circumstances like this. However, many of the chemotherapeutic protocols in use today are extremely toxic and may quickly destroy the patient's immune system and kill the patient as a consequence. And then we hear that old statement: "Well, the patient would have died anyway. We had to do something."

Some of the protocols used for advanced carcinoma of the colon in the past, for instance, were completely useless and should never have been considered in any treatment program for this disease.

The natural course of some of these conditions is never clearly understood because many aggressive physicians begin a treatment protocol even when there's no clear evidence that it helps.

The supervision the resident staff receives in University Medical Centers ranges from good to bad. When a patient tells his doctor that he feels like he's dying, the physician should listen attentively. It may turn out that the patient is only suffering from depression, which may be significant in itself. But in many cases, the patient really knows what he's talking about.

In Charlie's case, going home saved his life.

Chapter Thirty-two

From the Hills, the River

(Jacob's House)

The Tragic Chronicle of a Schizophrenic Doctor

~

*H*e felt the horse beneath him shake with tight muscles as he pounded down the road. He kept his head down and crouched lower, urging the horse on. He had to get to Jacob's House before the river overflowed its banks and caught him in its relentless onslaught. The rain kept falling from a sky that was black and gnarled with clouds moving rapidly and he heard its heavy rush in the air like a voice whispering. He didn't remember running out of the cabin into the wildness of the night, into the confusion of trembling leaves and wind, and he was almost surprised to find himself plunging through the darkness with the cold rain in his face. The rain stung him with its fierceness, forcing him to stay awake, but he still wasn't sure this wasn't all a dream. He didn't even remember running out to the barn and saddling the horse.

But he remembered the telephone, the mad insistent ringing in the night, and the voice, a whisper almost hissing, like the rain rushing, and sleep had broken in his tired mind into a thousand blurred fragments that fell apart and refused to arrange themselves in a coherent pattern.

"The River Road, Doctor," the voice hissed and he thought he could hear the rain through the receiver. "The last house...you know...Jacob's House. Oh please, please hurry for God's sake."

The words ran together, falling upon each other like the rain falling, a torrent of words that he was unable to decipher, like the river that was already flooding the muddy road. Yes, he thought,

Jacob's House, of course. And suddenly he was afraid. He felt his face hot with sweat and his throat tight and aching. Yes, Jacob's House, of course. But he couldn't remember what it was about Jacob's House that lay on the edge of his mind and gave him the curious feeling that he was reenacting something that was already long part of the past. He stood there puzzled, clenching the receiver tightly, watching the rain beat against the window and run down the glass, trying frantically to remember. He had the strange sensation of standing there holding the receiver and at the same time, as if from a distance, watching himself in his cabin, a ghost. This had never happened to him before and it frightened him.

Then he heard the desperate, urgent voice again, hissing into his ear, begging him to enter the violence of the night and forget the bewilderment of his own thoughts.

"You must come, Doctor, you must. Jacob is here and he...he's been hurt. Come quickly. I think he's dying."

It was a strange voice and yet oddly familiar, trembling with fear, broken and high, like a sound carried by the wind from far away and dying with a last soft prolonged murmur. Before he could fully understand the words, the wire went dead, the voice was gone, and he stood there for a while listening to the hum of the telephone and the wind outside weeping through the trees. The rain beating against his mind was a sharp splattering rhythm that made him ache to remember. Jumbled images and words totally dissociated from any organized arrangement raced through his distraught brain. He felt completely confused. He held his breath as he sensed the blackness all about him, moving, wet, cold, filled with something ominous from the past that he realized was drawing nearer, like his own shadow from which he could not escape.

Now he was on the road and he couldn't remember how he had gotten there. He couldn't understand what he was doing in the middle of that desolation, but somehow he was aware he had to go to the end of the road where Jacob's House was waiting for him; a rendezvous with an event that seemed as inevitable as death. He looked at the river, at its dark surface moving beneath the rain. He heard its dull swollen strength, rushing towards him from a time long since buried beneath the various events of his life, catching him with its swiftness, its terrible urgency, its coarse tumultuous fury.

For seven days the rain had come down and for seven days he had watched the river steadily inch up the banks, eating into the soft dirt and tugging at the roots of the trees there until they leaned over the water like tired old men, finally yielding to the swift currents and toppling into the roiling blackness that continued to swell.

"Hurry, Doctor, oh my God," he heard the voice again hissing into his ear. For the first time he wondered how anyone had known he was at his cabin. He was exhausted from long hours at the laboratory and desperately needed a rest. Only Ellen and his assistant Hendricks knew where he had gone. As he thought of Ellen and Hendricks he laughed quickly in the darkness with deliberate mirth. He felt the hot sweat of the horse and the cold rain on his body and he laughed again savagely and contemptuously. He heard himself above the rain and the swollen river and the drumming of the horse's hoofs on the muddy road. What a fool he had been, a fool, a tired fool, tired, old, a fool. Again he could see himself standing apart, a great distance away, safe, secluded, warm, dry, watching his other self, this pitiful old man whom he almost despised, riding through the night on his horse, while the rain pricked an icy tattoo on his face.

~

*H*e saw Ellen sitting across from him with her legs drawn up and her robe partly open, revealing white skin softly shadowed. She held her head back against the chair, her neck a beautiful gentle curve, her eyes nearly shut. He closed the book he had been reading and she looked at him. He saw her short dark hair mussed and curling about her forehead and he suddenly felt very old.

"You have a new assistant," she said, still looking at him intently.

"Yes," he said. "John Hendricks."

"You never told me," she said.

"I didn't think it would interest you. There are many administrative details, my dear, that are best left where they belong—at the laboratory."

"But daddy, after all, an assistant is something more than an administrative detail."

She frowned.

"I suppose you're right," he said, looking at the thick veins and the pigmented areas on the back of his hand.

He picked up his book but knew she was still looking at him. He didn't start reading, waiting for her to speak again.

She laughed softly, a sweet sound from deep in her throat.

"I actually think you're jealous already and I haven't even met the man."

She got up slowly with a long stretch and yawned like a sleepy young animal, bending over from the waist for a moment, as if waiting for him to get the full effect of the robe falling away from the soft swelling of her breasts. Superb choreography, he thought, instinctively performed. He had the uneasy feeling that she watched him carefully for any change in his expression. She then walked slowly and with deliberate grace, flat-bellied and long legged, in front of him.

He went back to examining his hand, almost being able to count the years he saw imprinted there.

"Has he been doing research long?"

"No. About a year, I guess."

She yawned again, softly, delicately, her lips parted slightly, her chest rising, ending with a long sigh like a partially suppressed musical sound deep in her throat. The sweet melody of youth, he thought.

"I wonder what makes a young man devote himself to research?" she said, mussing up her hair.

Shadows, he thought, shadows, energies from unknown sources directing you while you think you alone are plotting your destiny.

"A man of twenty-eight, my dear," he said, "is prepared for serious work."

He turned back to his book but still felt she was looking at him. He read a page without absorbing one word, turned it and then turned it back again, rereading it without the slightest comprehension. He then closed the book in total surrender.

"What were you doing when you were twenty-eight, daddy?"

She sounded like a child asking her father a silly question. Calling him "daddy" made him feel ancient. Thirty-two years fled in his mind like a rapidly rewinding video and he thought thirty-two years, thirty-two years, thirty-two years. He sighed.

"Now don't get angry with me, daddy," she said.

"I am not angry with you, dear," he said, but he knew his voice was too loud and sharp.

He looked at the book in his lap, flipped it open once again in total futility, and then slammed it shut.

"I was in research," he said, his voice soft again but betraying his over-control by its measured cadence, each word marching out of his mouth as though in single file. "Old men doing research were once young men doing research."

She came over to him, continuing to perform her beautifully choreographed ballet.

"Of course, daddy. I'm sorry. I didn't mean to upset you."

She brushed her hand against his cheek, bending from the waist to kiss him, again showing him the soft swelling of her breasts. She walked toward the bedroom then, with the smooth deliberate steps of a dancer walking off stage.

"Invite him to dinner, won't you, daddy?" she said, turning her head so that her lips were near the gentle hollow of her shoulder.

"I shall if you want me to."

"It's only proper, daddy. After all, he is your assistant."

"Yes, he is," he said.

He watched her disappear into the bedroom and then picked up his book. He knew it would be useless to follow her.

Thirty-two years, he thought.

As he sat in the chair, he gradually became aware that he was observing himself sitting there. It was from a great distance, as if from space. But he also knew that while sitting there he couldn't observe this other self who was watching him from space. It became difficult for him, at first, to detect who was his real self, the person sitting so peacefully in the chair or the being who watched him from space. After some moments, however, he realized that the figure sitting in the easy chair was merely an illusion. He was convinced of this when the individual in the chair began to disintegrate before his very eyes. His flesh fell off in huge chunks leaving the bones exposed. Then everything fell apart, and he watched as his dislocated pile of bones, skin, organs, and blood scattered infinitely in all directions in his own private universe, while he did nothing but observe this panorama like a totally disinterested traveler who just happened to be standing on a corner in space, bewildered and unable to comprehend intelligently the complete dispersion of his own soul.

~

*J*ack Hendricks was placed on this earth for only one purpose, to please women. That was his firm belief. His mind was occupied with this thought twenty-four hours a day. He believed that he had his first erection while still in utero at three months gestation. There was only one group of women he couldn't please and that was the radical feminists. According to Jack, these women felt that nobody should be that beautiful and have two over-functioning testicles as a bonus.

Jack was always in splendid attire. His clothes were expensive, bought with money that was lavishly bestowed upon him by his doting father, a corporate attorney in Boston. And Jack had the kind of body that made everything he wore look great. He was six feet two inches tall, weighed one hundred eighty pounds, all muscle and bone kept in a constant state of perfection by daily exercise. With his well-combed dark hair, a thick trim beard, light skin, and blue eyes, he had all the physical attributes of a devilishly handsome actor.

He was intelligent but not brilliant. He started out as an internist but gave that up because of the work-load, low compensation, and erratic hours, a life style that prevented him from fulfilling his purpose on this planet. When the position as Dr. Honicutt's assistant was offered to him, a situation somehow miraculously arranged by his father, he was shocked but accepted it immediately. The idea of regular hours and every weekend off was appealing. After he met Dr. Honicutt's young wife, Ellen, he was absolutely sure that he had made the right decision. On initial eye contact, he was immediately aware of the infinite possibilities regarding their relationship. He figured it was only a matter of time. When Ellen suggested that the three of them have lunch together, Jack knew this was the beginning of another conquest. He looked forward to it with great anticipation.

~

*I*t was a dark, gloomy day with threatening clouds overhead when Sorina awoke on the front steps of Jacob's House. Old Jacob heard something thump on the front porch. He grabbed his shotgun and went to investigate.

"Who are you?" he asked, standing over her scowling. He thought, at first, she was a drunk who had been dumped there by her boyfriend.

"My name is Sorina."

She wore a brilliant red headdress with dangling silver disks. A necklace of gold medals hung around her neck. Gold bracelets jangled from her wrists as she tried to sit up straight. There were rings on all her fingers, with a variety of semiprecious stones. With her glistening black hair, thick as a horse's tail, dark eyes and swarthy skin, she was undoubtedly a gypsy, Jacob thought. A group of them had been seen wandering through the area recently.

"Why are you here?" he asked impatiently. "And where did you come from?"

"I come from the Carpathian Mountains in Rumania, from a people doomed to wander forever," she said. "But why I am here, I do not know."

She shrugged her shoulders and then winced as she touched the side of her head.

"All I remember is that I have walked a great distance for many days and I find myself suddenly here at your doorstep. But again I cannot answer why exactly here on this spot. I know that I must be here for some purpose. What that purpose is, however, I will have to wait and see. I have seen enough of life to know that nothing happens by accident in this world."

"You can't stay here," Jacob said, holding the gun under his right arm.

"I am going, do not worry, my dear friend, I am going," Sorina said.

She pushed herself up to a standing position with great difficulty, staggered for a few moments, and then collapsed into Jacob's arms.

"Damn," he yelled out. "Who needs this?"

He carried her into the house and stretched her out on the couch. She was moaning. He felt her head. There was a large bump just above her left ear. When he touched it, she groaned with pain. He removed her kerchief and applied a cold wet pack to the side of her head. He took out a small flashlight from a black leather bag in the closet and lifting her eyelids, checked the reaction of her pupils. They were equal and normally reactive. He let out a long sigh. He pulled a chair over to the couch and sat down, watching her suspiciously. It took about ten minutes for her to regain consciousness.

She opened her eyes. She was frightened and breathed rapidly. The cold pack slipped off her head as she tried to sit up. She fell back groaning.

"Don't move," Jacob said. "You're still too weak."

He reapplied the pack.

"You have a nasty lump above your left ear," he said.

She groaned and closed her eyes.

"I am truly sorry to cause you this trouble," Sorina said softly, her voice barely audible. "I shall be on my way soon. Do not worry."

"You understand," Jacob said, still looking at her suspiciously, "that I am not a 'gajo,' an easy prey, as you people say."

"Rom san tu?" Sorina looked up quickly. "You are a gypsy?"

"No, but gypsies have been through here before and I don't plan to be robbed," Jacob said, his eyes narrowing.

"Ah," Sorina groaned again, holding her head. "Forgive me, but you speak like a fool. All gypsies do not steal. I will leave now and then you can stop worrying."

She tried to get up but fell back again.

"You must lie there quietly. If you prefer, I will call the police and they can take you to the hospital ten miles from here."

"No police, I beg of you," Sorina cried out quickly, her eyes flashing. "Gypsies and police do not mix well."

"It's five miles into town and too far to walk in your condition. As you can see, a storm is threatening and it will soon be raining. You will stay here. You've had a concussion but there is no fracture."

"Are you a man of medicine?" Sorina asked.

"Yes," Jacob answered.

He turned and looked up suddenly at a young woman standing on the stairs.

"Go back to your room," he yelled out harshly, his eyes flaming. "And don't come out until I tell you. You will nurse that bastard child of yours now just as I instructed you to do."

Sorina turned just in time to see a slender, pale, young woman ascend the stairs silently.

"Your daughter, Doctor?" she asked.

"My wife, my heartache, and my mistake," Jacob answered fiercely.

The rain came suddenly with a wild rush.

It rained for three days and Sorina could hear the menacing sound of the river as it began to overflow its banks. Every night she heard the violent arguments between the old doctor and his young wife, as intense as the storm outside. Sorina would leave the room and stand on the landing, fear in her heart. Words like "bitch" and "whore" floated up to her as she stood there trembling. She was caught between the storm, the river, and the uncontrolled vehemence of the old doctor. She wondered what mysterious forces had been unleashed to lead her to this house by the river.

The storm was not letting up.

On the third night, she heard Jacob threaten his wife with a horsewhipping. The young woman laughed derisively and Sorina shook her head and sucked in her breath.

"You wouldn't dare, you old cockroach."

Sorina heard the loud snap of the whip followed by a piercing scream.

"Don't, you're choking me," the young woman screamed again. The scream seemed to last forever and then stopped suddenly, ending in a terrible sucking sound.

Sorina then realized why she had come to this house. She returned hurriedly to her room. She snatched a raincoat and hat from the closet and ran quickly to the baby's room. He was sound asleep. She bundled him up and slipped him inside the raincoat against her chest. Her heart was pounding. She was about to descend the stairs when she heard Jacob coming up. She closed her bedroom door without making a sound. She heard him walk to her door, his heavy breathing making her think a wild beast was ready to attack. Sorina held her breath, praying silently that the baby would not wake up. The baby moved gently beneath the raincoat. She heard Jacob walk to the baby's room. She quickly slipped out of her room and descended the stairs soundlessly. As she opened the front door and stepped out into the wild turbulence of the storm, she heard Jacob's heavy footsteps cross quickly to her room. He was yelling at the top of his voice.

"Where are you, you gypsy whore? What have you done with that bastard child?"

She was already down the road when she heard him kick open the front door and shoot his gun three times into the darkness of the heavens.

~

Alex Honicutt had graduated from medical school at the age of twenty-eight and got his first job with Langley in Chicago, the internationally known researcher whose work on the kidney had taken medicine out of the dark ages. Alex had nothing more to his credit than a summa cum laude and the intense anxiety to prove himself. But yet, in a way, he was in no hurry. He believed destiny had chosen him for greatness and with rigid self-discipline, only time was necessary to achieve his goals. He held a fixed idea of the type of mind needed for research in the basic sciences and felt signally qualified for the role. He convinced himself that a controlled, relentless driving force was necessary for all great accomplishments; that inexorable push whipping the flesh when it begins to flag and relax, tempered by flashes of intuitive imagination, an ability to seize upon a chance combination of events and extract a wholly new idea, never before conceived by any other human being on this earth. That was the ultimate thrill and excitement in unraveling the secrets of the human body.

He was all alone in the world. The death of his mother and father had been sequestered in the deepest recesses of his mind. He remembered the old gypsy woman who had raised him from infancy telling him an awful tale of death and calamity regarding his parents. He never thought or spoke about them from that moment.. Being alone and feeling alone made him ideally suited for a life of solitude in research, an existence stripped of all emotion with only the squealing and grunting of the animals to keep him company.

His apparently limitless energies drove him forward, an inner agitation preventing him from relaxing and enjoying the simple spontaneous, totally disorganized activities of young people. He was a dedicated loner. Early in his life he had made the vow that each day he would work as if it were his last, and yet lay plans as if death were some fantastic impossibility.

He spent ten years with Langley, working on the various phases of kidney function. He considered this his apprenticeship. Even there he didn't deny his pride in his work, his recognition of his own abilities, his own genius, although he worked in the shadow of one of the greatest contributors to medical knowledge of this century. As a man grows, he thought, so does the concept of himself grow; and this concept is the matrix that shapes his destiny. His destiny was greatness and he accepted it without question.

One day Dr. Langley came up to him in the lab and put his arm around his shoulders.

"Alex," Dr. Langley said, "I want you to know how much we've appreciated your work here. But now I think you're ready for the next phase of your life. Adolf Moench in Vienna called me yesterday, asking for help in finding a new assistant. You'll be working with a modern day Pasteur on all the complex phases of water and electrolyte balance that I'm sure will ultimately lead to a dialyzer, the artificial kidney that I know is the goal of your work."

Alex didn't have to think twice. He was on the plane the next day. Moench, himself, was at the airport to pick him up. Alex recognized him immediately, having attended several of his lectures. He looked like a little dried-up vegetable with a ragged mustache that drooped on one side.

The trip to the apartment that Moench had already engaged for him was harrowing. Moench kept up a steady stream of small talk while driving through red lights and stop signs, totally oblivious of the other traffic. He left a trail of vitriol hurled out of windows of countless automobiles amidst the high pitched squealing of tires as frustrated and maddened drivers slammed on their brakes.

He would never forget that tender old man who walked carefully turned to the right to compensate for a slightly lurching gait to the left. Every summer the old man grew his beautiful tomato plants in boxes hanging outside the laboratory windows. Besides his lurch, and his general unsteadiness that gave him the appearance that he was about to fall, he made matters worse by neglecting to tie his sneakers, which were always a part of his uniform of the day. His fly was generally open and when Alex brought this to his attention the first week he was there, Moench stopped and looked down for a moment.

"Alex," he said, like an old school teacher, "remember one of the fundamental rules of the universe: what can't get up, can't get out."

Moench always wore the same tattered blue sweater with holes in both elbows. His brain would have stopped functioning without it. When he was about to write a new article on mammalian kidney function that would set the medical world on fire, his eyes would gleam with an intensity and excitement that was immediately infectious. After working endless hours on some phase of renal function to clarify a point, he would stop suddenly, throw his lab coat to the floor, grab Alex by the arm and propel him hurriedly towards the door.

"The brain is drunk with work. We must sober it up immediately with some good dark Austrian beer or it will begin to malfunction from dehydration."

He'd keep muttering under his breath, humming snatches of Strauss's Die Fledermaus while he scurried along.

Alex often felt annoyed by these diversions from laboratory routine, but they'd be off, the old man holding him by the elbow and steering him to the street.

They'd enter the cool darkness of the rathskeller around the corner and Moench would yell out to the attractive, plump, heavy-breasted woman behind the counter: "Anna, we are here to sober up. Please hurry with the beer and bratwurst and radish and some of that magnificent dark bread you bake with your special magic."

"What are you, Dr. Moench, the King of Sweden with all your orders?" Anna would reply with a big smile and everybody would laugh.

The rest of the day would be gone as they sat for hours with tall sweating mugs of cold dark beer, the old man's mustache wet and drooping with foam. They'd talk of the sky, the sea, the mountains, the sadness and happiness of men and women, and the grand illusion that was called life. The more the beer flowed, the more philosophy poured out of Moench. During one of those sessions when the old man had much more than his usual share of beer, he looked at Alex, all the while tugging at his elbow to maintain his attention.

"You know, Alex, there's not much difference between a man and a river," he said. "A man, like a river, begins in the hills, in the voluptuous roundness of his mother. He surges forward into this world gathering speed, ripping at the banks that hold him in and control his course. At times, he will overflow the banks and destroy everything in his path. At other times, he will reach a quiet pool where he will take stock of himself and his position in the world. And then he'll be on his way again, mindless of the destruction he may leave in his path as he rushes to reach his own particular private ocean. He usually forgets that in the process of destroying others, he destroys himself."

The old man had looked so strangely at Alex then and for such a long time that Alex turned away, his face on fire.

"Anna," the old man called out.

"Yes, your highness," Anna yelled back, trotting over immediately.

"Give my young friend, Alex, a big hug and one of your big smothering kisses, just to let him know what it feels like to be kissed and hugged by a real Austrian woman who happens to be endowed by nature so monumentally."

Before Alex could do or say anything, his face was pressed against her huge bosom and held there until he thought he would suffocate. This maneuver was then followed by a big wet kiss on the lips.

"Now we are ready for more beer, Anna," the old man said as Alex sat there still gasping for air.

Much as Alex admired Moench, he did not overlook his faults. He felt that if Moench had restricted himself to the rigid self-discipline of the laboratory and drove himself harder, the world would have been astounded by his prolific genius. There was no doubt that he could have been another Pasteur, but too much beer and philosophy had weakened the matrix.

During one of their frequent visits to Anna's rathskeller, the plump, smiling lady waltzed over and said, "Come with me, Alex, to the kitchen. I want you to meet my little gem. And you, old man, you sit there and drink your beer while the young ones meet."

In the kitchen was an angel of indescribable beauty and innocence, blond and blue-eyed.

"This is my niece from Steyr, Liesalotte Krantz, Alex, the joy of my heart. She is going to work here for the summer, having just completed her studies at the university. Her real work will begin in September in Salzburg in computers. Please sit down and talk to each other while I go about my business."

Anna whisked away and left them standing there, each attempting to start a conversation, embarrassed, and finally laughing as they sat down over kaffe and kuchen.

From that moment, Alex's life took an abrupt turn. He was swept away from the sterile atmosphere of the lab to a love in full flower with concerts, dances, parties, and hikes through the mountains. It revealed a side to his personality that he didn't know existed.

"Vienna is the city of love and music," Liesa said, breathless just at the thought of it. "It's the city of Mozart, Beethoven, Brahms, and Schubert. I shall show you everything that excites me. We'll start with Wurstelprater, our famous amusement park with its giant ferris wheel, the Riesenrad. We'll visit Schonbrunn Palace, where our imperial family lived for more than two hundred years, and where Napoleon was nearly assassinated. You must see St. Stephen's Cathedral on Stephenplatz. We'll do some shopping in the elegant shops on Kartner Strasse. Next will be Mozart's home on Singerstrasse where he composed his opera Figaro. I know that you'll want to visit Sigmund Freud's home at 19 Berggasse in the 9th District, being a physician yourself. In between these interesting places, we'll stop and have kaffe and taste our famous sachertorte."

She hugged and kissed him.

"Oh, Alex, I'm so happy."

~

While they were having kaffe one day, enjoying the warmth of the spring day, sitting in their favorite coffee shop and watching the people go by, Liesa turned to him and said out of the blue, "Tell me about your mother and father."

It was like a blow to the head, at first, to hear that question that he dreaded so much. He had never mentioned his parents or his past to anyone before. When pressed, he would laugh and say, "I'm a child of the wind that blows from the mountains and streams, a free spirit raised by an old gypsy woman doomed to wander the globe forever, who taught me to worship the sun and the moon, the stars that Van Gogh painted into the heavens, how to harness the solar wind and the burning fire within me, to recognize and utilize the good and evil spirits, fairies, elves, and vampires. I am a strange and lonely boy."

The subject would change and Alex would be off the hook.

With Liesa, he opened up and told her everything, completely surprising himself.

Up to the age of sixteen, he accepted Sorina as his mother. At that time she told him how she had collapsed on the front steps of his father's house from a concussion that she couldn't remember sustaining; and standing at the top of the stairs, listening in the darkness as his father strangled his mother because he thought Alex wasn't his child; and finally rushing out into the fury of the night to escape the deadly wrath of the old man, learning later of his death.

Little by little Sorina taught Alex the ways of the gypsy, introducing him to the astounding world of magic with special chants, incantations, and spells.

She told him about the cauldron, a magical container which originally was used to collect blood from human sacrifices, but now was merely a symbol of eternal life. She explained the significance of the magic circle, nine feet in diameter, with another smaller circle eight feet in diameter inside. In between the two circles are inscribed crosses, names of powers and magical herbs, such as vervain, which thwart the desires of the demons. She demonstrated how a small gap is made in the circles to allow the magician in. The gap must be closed immediately upon the magician's entrance to prevent evil forces from following and harming the magician.

Inside the inner circle, the magician faces east and makes the sign of the equal-armed cross which represents the four elements, the four principal points, and mastery of all things on this earth. He clasps an imaginary sword and vibrates with the frightening force of God. Then, clapping his hands above his head, the magician intones, "May the almighty archangel Rafael protect me from all the evil approaching from the east." The same ritual is repeated facing south, speaking to the archangel Michael, west to the archangel Gabriel, and north to the archangel Uriel.

The awesome infusion of power into the body of the magician can influence another person's subconscious mind, causing him to become subservient to the magician. However, one must never forget that the main purpose of this ritual is, basically, to use the laws of nature through the power of the will.

Alex could still hear Sorina's voice as she repeated, "Magic is used to develop a person's subconscious powers to such a level that will permit him to overcome all obstacles in his life, so that he may enjoy his brief sojourn on this planet to the fullest extent."

There are four main laws of magic, Sorina explained: "To know, to dare, to will, to keep silent."

Some people are gifted with natural psychic power and Sorina felt Alex was one of those.

"You must learn to concentrate your power effectively to practice magic properly," Sorina said. "And this power is based on the natural laws of the universe. If you contrive to break a natural law, you will then suffer a total spiritual disintegration."

This raw energy is released from the deep recesses of the subconscious mind and reveals itself as the basic instincts, which are the will to live, to beget, and the herding instinct, which all animals have. Some philosophers believe there is a fourth instinct that raises man above the animals, the religious force, the balancing force that permits an individual to control his more primitive urges.

While Alex was still an infant, Sorina performed magical rituals over him which ensured his future greatness.

He was also taught never to point at a rainbow; that a treasure lay beneath the spot where the first swallow is seen each spring; if he met a woman with an empty jug, it was a bad omen; if a horse's skull is placed on the front gate, ghosts refuse to enter; if you collect the yellow roots of the gandergoose plant in the dark on Easter, and crush them, mixing in a few drops of your own blood, finally blending a small amount of this concoction in the food of the woman you love, she in turn will love you and remain forever faithful. For a barren woman, Sorina had a special stone which she would scrape, mixing the dust-like particles with pure water; the resultant mixture when drunk would cause the barren woman to become pregnant immediately, even if her husband had not slept with her for years.

Sorina warned Alex against the evil eye and revealed the secrets that would protect him. For wounds, she used plantain or mallow; for liver ailments, dandelion and hops; for coughs, coltsfoot; and for fevers, yarrow and sorrel.

Alex begged her to tell him his fortune by using tea leaves, reading his palm, or using Tarot cards. She refused all his requests.

"Looking into the future," she would say solemnly, "can destroy your present happiness, Alex. Live your future a day at a time."

~

While he was in this maddeningly heightened flush of love, his mind constantly full of images of his angelic Liesa, the gentle curve of her cheeks, her nose, her lips, her ears, her neck, he began to have sudden urges to pull away by himself, to withdraw into the shadows. He began to wonder if everybody looked at him with a strange and questioning glance.

One night after working at the lab until late in the evening, he came back to his apartment in complete exhaustion. He sat down in his favorite easy chair, staring at the lamp across the room. He stared at it for over an hour and the lamp gradually changed. It was no longer just a simple lamp. It appeared to have a life of its own, existing independently without any relationship to its form and function. While he continued to stare at it with greater and greater intensity, it began to fragment, separating into many pieces, each piece hanging in the air by some invisible wire. Then a flood of thoughts rushed through his mind, so rapidly he was unable to identify any of them. He felt himself in a heightened state of superconsciousness associated with a disordered sense of unreality. He gradually entered a dangerous, threatening, alien world, with a central, bright, glaring, overpowering light. He became totally unaware of the passage of time, sitting there immobilized until dawn. He recognized immediately that he was in the grasp of absolute truth, the ultimate, a strange zone that was timeless, where he stood at the side of God.

That day everything continued to appear strange. Dr. Moench spoke to him, his face distorted as if by a faulty lens in a camera, his voice separated from the motion of his lips, his eyes probing questioningly. Alex understood everything that was said to him but he realized at the same time that he was still in the alien world he had entered the night before. Everything seemed shrouded in absurdity and incongruity. When he came back to his apartment that evening, he walked back and forth laughing at the top of his voice for a long time. He felt as if some being from another universe had taken command of his mind. He tried to sleep but he heard voices in the walls. They spoke to him but wordlessly. He thought if not with words, then with what? With music? No, not with music. With sounds, yes, with sounds stripped of their relationships to objects, a pure language that was at once understandable and not understandable. He would suddenly sit up in bed, his whole body feeling encased in steel but yet moving uneasily with the slow athetoid motions of an individual afflicted with cerebral palsy. At the same time, thoughts flooded through his mind endlessly, so rapidly he couldn't grasp their meaning.

The next morning, he didn't get out of bed, his eyes shut tightly against the light of day. Suddenly, he realized Moench was leaning over him.

"Alex, Alex," Moench kept repeating. "Are you ill?"

"No, I am not ill, Dr. Moench," Alex replied.

"Then why aren't you up and in the laboratory?"

"I really don't know the answer to that question, Dr. Moench, so it's useless to ask the question. But I do know that I am not ill. Please let me lie here for a while. I shall arrive at the lab in due time. Thank you for coming."

Alex didn't open his eyes to look at the old man.

Moench stood there for a few minutes, not knowing whether to leave or just sit and watch.

"You may leave, Dr. Moench," Alex said finally. "I assure you there is nothing wrong."

Dr. Moench turned and left, feeling uneasy.

At mid-afternoon, Moench was busy catching up on his lab notes when Alex walked in.

"Alex," Dr. Moench said, "I'm so glad to see you back in the laboratory."

"Thank you, Dr. Moench. I'm ready for work like I said I would be. I'll catch up on my notes first just as you appear to be doing."

He saw the questioning look in Moench's eyes. How could he discuss something with the old doctor that he himself didn't understand or was too frightened to think about?

Over the next few weeks, every evening on arriving at his apartment, he made it a ritual to sit in his easy chair and stare at the lamp. Nothing happened. There was no aura ("trema"), no "truth-taking stare" ("die wahrnehmungstarre"), no "stimmung," the emotional response that is associated with the stare, no disturbance of any kind that gave him that frightening sense of unreality. He was not transported to that spectacular alien world. There was no torrent of thoughts flying through his mind with an impossible speed, no "bright dazzling light," no intense awareness of absolute truth. There was no jubilation as he had previously experienced when he had felt he was standing at the right hand of God.

The lamp did not fragment and for that he was grateful. He knew enough psychiatry to suspect that he had experienced a brief psychotic break. He remembered what Dr. Phillip Downs, the chief of psychiatry, had told his fourth-year class in medical school: "The more sudden the break, the more sudden the recovery."

He was now haunted by the fear that schizophrenia would rob him of his life-long ambition to discover the ultimate secrets of the kidney that would lead to the development of a small portable dialyzing unit.

He again buried himself in his work, seeing Liesa only infrequently. Their few hours together were a form of play-acting and totally without any emotional involvement on his part.

Finally, the day before Liesa's departure for Salzburg arrived. He had promised to spend the entire day with her as a final, though, temporary, farewell. It was mid-September and the morning air was crisp and cool. They met for a light breakfast and dressed in lederhosen, started out on a hiking path in the hills outside the city.

"I come here often to hike," Liesa said quietly when they sat down to rest. "This is where I think great thoughts."

"About what," Alex said smiling, amused by the serious tone of her voice.

"About life and death," Liesa said. "About my place on this earth. To submerge myself in, I suppose you could call it, pantheism."

"Pantheism?" Alex said surprised. "Those are truly great thoughts, Liesa. I never suspected that you would think of yourself as a pantheist."

"I majored in computers, Alex, but my minor was philosophy. You know very little about me and I know even less about you."

Liesa stood up, ready to go.

"We had a good start at the beginning in getting to know each other," Liesa said, a sad note in her voice, "but something happened that I don't really understand."

"Neither do I," Alex said, "but we shouldn't let that stop us from enjoying the present moment together."

They climbed a steep ridge overlooking the valley. Down below, a stream wandered haphazardly through fields as far as they could see. The sun was bright and it was warmer than when they had started the hike. They were on a section of the hiking trail with a sharp drop of a hundred feet when they stopped for Liesa to take off her sweater. Alex could see the jagged rocks far below.

They were very close together when Alex first heard the voice.

"Push Liesa off the path," it said.

The voice was so loud that Alex jerked up suddenly at the sound, bumping into Liesa. She dropped to her knees as she lost her footing and began to slide off the narrow path. She grabbed at his ankles and he began to slide with her. He took hold of a small sapling growing out of the side of the hill and with his other hand managed to pull her back to the path.

Liesa began to shudder. She cried against his shoulder as they held each other tightly.

"You fool," the voice said, "push her off the path. I order you to push her off."

"No," Alex said loudly. "I will not."

Liesa looked up at him.

"What is it, Alex?" she said, still sobbing.

"It's nothing, Liesa, really nothing. I just wrenched my leg and it nearly gave way when I pulled you back."

"You were talking to your leg, Alex?"

"Yes, I was talking to my leg."

They both started to laugh. They kissed.

That night they slept together.

The next morning at the train station, Alex felt like a robot. He felt no emotion as Liesa stood crying on the train platform next to him. He kissed her on the cheek and promised to see her as soon as he could get some time off. Anna didn't speak to him. It was all over in a few minutes. Liesa was gone and Alex returned to the laboratory feeling dead.

That night he sat in his favorite chair and stared at his magic lamp. There was no fragmentation and he didn't enter his alien world. He read for several hours. He felt an odd exhilaration that kept him from sleeping. When the clock struck midnight, he went downstairs and drove to the redlight district. The ladies of the night were out in full force. He pulled over to the curb at a darkened corner. He saw a woman approach the car.

"Get in," he said.

He drove down by the river and parked.

"Now! Do it now!" an insistent voice whispered in his head.

He put his hands on the whore's neck with both thumbs on her larynx and squeezed hard until he heard the snap. He did it so quickly she hadn't had time to resist. She slumped over, gasping and wheezing with a horrible sucking sound. He looked up and down the street. It was empty. He pulled her out of the car and dumped her into the river. He stood at the river's edge, watching as she floated with the current for a few seconds and then slipped beneath the surface.

He drove back to his apartment and fell asleep as soon as he hit the bed.

One week later, he packed his bags, said good-bye to a startled Dr. Moench, and caught a flight back to the United States.

~

*L*ightning tore the savage blackness and everything leaped out of the night at him, the trees stretching their gauntness over the road, their stormy branches moving with agonizing awkwardness. The sharp cracking of thunder followed and the horse with ears stiff, swerved suddenly and he nearly slipped from the wet saddle. As the horse continued to heave, he remembered with a vague uneasiness what Moench had said years ago, beer dripping from his mustache: "...in destroying others, destroys himself," and he wondered if Moench had intuitively suspected something about Alex even then.

He heard the voice over the telephone again, hissing into his ear and he was afraid of the lightning and the thunder and the swollen river that ate into the soft banks and pulled down the trees, hungry, writhing, black. He wanted to turn back but the road behind him was ugly with the skeletal limbs of bare and lonely trees extended in a deathly embrace. He bent down lower until he could feel his elbows on the horse and the smell of the rain-soaked sweating animal was strong in his nostrils.

He felt now that he must be dreaming, but the rain roared in his ears and he shivered with the cold. He looked up at the sky. It was like blackened smudged glass. It moved with him, pressing down on him. He caught his tongue between his teeth and the pain shot in his mouth. The wind increased in intensity, whipping the rain against him in ferocious gusts. He heard the loud clattering of the trees as they joined the wind in a macabre dance.

~

Alex had gotten a job with a big pharmaceutical company in Connecticut on his return to the states. He was given his own lab where he could do what he wanted. Ten years slipped by quickly as he involved himself in his work. He had buried the magic lamp deep in his brain, along with the whore in Vienna. But the thought of Liesa nagged at him relentlessly. He finally took a two-week vacation and caught a flight to Salzburg. He called the lab in Vienna from the airport. He was told by the secretary that Moench had died the previous December. The secretary knew Anna and Liesa. Alex managed to wrangle Liesa's address from her. Liesa was working for Monitor Computers in Salzburg.

Alex parked across the street from the main entrance. A narrow park with benches and trees separated the two lanes of traffic. He sat in the car and stared at the entrance to the building. Two hours later, he saw Liesa walk out. She was just as beautiful as ever. He ran across the street and walked behind her. She stopped at the intersection and looked back. Her eyes widened. She stood there looking at him, unable to believe her eyes.

"Alex," she said finally, a tone of anger in her voice. "What do you want from me?"

"I just wanted to see you once again, Liesa. I happened to be in the area on business."

She stood in front of him silently, unmoving.

"Now you've seen me, Alex. You've satisfied your curiosity. Now what?"

She was abrupt and cold.

Alex hesitated. He realized this encounter would lead to nothing.

"I thought that perhaps...," he stammered, waited, and then continued. "Perhaps you'd have a glass of wine or a cup of coffee with me before I fly back to the States."

She waited a moment on the edge of refusing but then surrendered.

While sipping her wine, she looked directly at Alex.

"Why did you run away, Alex?"

"That's a question I'll never be able to answer, Liesa. I don't know. Intelligent people often do stupid things and I've regretted it deeply."

She told him that she had married an electrical engineer about two years after Alex had left and that she had a son ten years old.

"Ten years old?" Alex said surprised, suddenly realizing what she was telling him.

"Yes, ten years old," Liesa said. "He is your son, Alex, but I'm not going to allow you to interfere with our lives in any way. You understand? My husband is a fine man who is raising the boy as his own. And when you leave here, I want you to forget about me, the boy, and everything that we once meant to each other."

She stood up suddenly and walked out, leaving him sitting there, unable to speak.

~

Alex thought of Hendricks and his face contorted. His hands tightened on the reins until they were stiff and aching. He saw the young face smiling, the straight white teeth, the tight muscles, and he remembered the thirty-two years. Thirty-two years of working late into the night alone with his rats, frogs, dogs, and cats, imprisoned behind thick walls of solitude, always fearful that some night he would come home, sit down to relax and suddenly stare at the lamp on the table and see it begin to fragment.

As he neared the age of sixty, his loneliness deepened and he became aware of a gradual change within him. The last few years brought a weariness, a fatigue, not only of the body, with which he had been able to cope previously, but also of the spirit. This he repressed by driving his flagging mind with a renewed but dwindling intensity. His exhaustion grew and no longer did the genius of his mind seize and congeal the elements of the laboratory into useful concepts.

A fear began to grow within him that he wouldn't be able to finish his work on the dialyzer. Each day this fear underwent a mitosis like a slow-growing malignancy, reproducing and increasing in strength, invading his brain and robbing him of the power he needed to continue his work.

He thought of a long vacation, a trip to some distant land, a change of scenery; something that would transfuse his body with its former drive, its familiar fierce, unrelenting force. He thought of Liesa and Austria and the son he had never seen, but immediately ruled it out. Not just because of the frozen reception he would have received from Liesa. The magic lamp and the final fragmentation of his soul stared him in the face. He knew eventually that he wouldn't be able to escape from that alien world that threatened to engulf him. For now, though, he still had some serious work to complete.

While he groped for new inspiration, the fear of a total mental blockade grew into horrible proportions, further dulling his senses.

His energies, once so easily channelled into productive work, gradually lessened and what little remained flew off in all directions.

~

*T*hen Ellen came and he felt a sudden release, an escape from the rigid discipline of his scientific mind. It was like an escape into the sun from a frigid isolation. Like Liesa, she had just graduated from the university, Harvard, at the top of her class. For Alex, it was déjà-vu. Was he getting a second chance in life to make up for the stupid mistakes he had made with Liesa?

He remembered that first warm day of spring with patches of snow scattered like tattered clouds on the hills. The sun was bright. They walked a short distance out of town, along an old Indian trail next to the river, out among the trees with their shadows running from the old roots exposed on the drying ground. The air was sparkling, clean, warm, and yet cool.

Ellen kept looking at him and smiling, her lips red and moist, her nose a little shiny, her eyes blue against her white skin and short dark hair. Every time he looked at her he felt an extreme happiness tinged with pain.

"What's the matter, Alex?" Ellen asked him.

"Nothing. I was just thinking."

"Of what?" She smiled and took hold of his hand. "Of the snow and how it melts in the spring?"

She laughed softly, a delicate musical sound. She was happy and pretty and pleased with herself and her youthful vitality. He felt old and tired.

"Or maybe you were thinking of the shadows and how they look like fallen trees that we can see but can't touch."

Yes, shadows, he thought. Weightless shadows we can't touch that rest on us heavily. Shadows that can crush us with their weightless heaviness.

He looked at her and smiled.

"I was thinking of you," he said. "And how much you've changed my life."

"Do I make you that sad?"

She brought her face close to his, her eyes wide. He smelled the perfume in her hair.

"Yes, you make me very sad," he said quietly, "but at the same time, very happy."

"I'm glad," she said.

He pulled her to his chest and kissed her on the lips. He felt the soft sweetness of her arms around him and her hands gently pressing on his back.

"You know I love you, Ellen," he said, his face against her hair.

She kissed him then, breathing quickly, her mouth open and hot. He could feel her breasts moving against him as he held her tightly to his chest. They stayed on the side of the hill until the sun went down, watching the shadows gradually stretching across the ground, while the clouds were like the soft belly feathers of some magnificent bird, glowing pink against the darkening sky.

He remembered the hills always, their softness curving into the shadows that darkened as he watched with Ellen, the pines plunging into the lengthening shadows and the gentle roundness of the hills. Moench was right. A man is like a river. He begins in the hills, emerging from the shadows, but forever destined to carry his shadows with him, no matter where he goes or what spectacular heights he attains.

~

*L*ightning ripped the heavens and he saw a house loom out of the blackness. It jutted against the night like some evil mansion, its chimney rising to the clouds. Suddenly he remembered the River Road. Only it had been the Bloody River Road at that time long ago. The night had been the same, tempestuous, with the wind whipping the rain through the trees, and the river threatening with its bloated strength. He remembered the house, too, Old Jacob's House it was called, the old house on River Road, the only house, and Old Jacob, the hermit, Old Jacob. The house had been partly torn down over the years by time and the elements. The only things left standing were the chimney and the gaping hole of the foundation, with crumbling bricks and rotting timbers.

Everybody had been surprised when Jacob got married to Martha Gormely. She was only twenty-two and had the reputation of sleeping in anybody's bed who asked her. The townspeople called Old Jacob an old fool. At the end of nine months she bore him a son and everybody in the village had a big laugh about guessing who the father was. And then Jacob strangled her the night of the violent storm when the river overflowed its banks. Bloody River Road, the good people called it after that. They fished Old Jacob out of the river the next day, his body torn by the rushing water that seemed as furious and savage as his own rage. The baby was never found. The river had gradually lost its strength and the house began to rot. For a while, the story floated around town that Jacob had given the baby to an old gypsy woman who believed in witchcraft. The surprising thing about the whole sad affair was that after her marriage to Jacob, nobody could get close to Martha Gormely. Not that some of the good men of the town didn't try. It was whispered that she had gotten religious.

Alex heard the sound of the soil being eaten away, slipping into the swift current like Old Jacob's body and carried away through the blackness. He saw Martha, Jacob's young wife, with her head twisted oddly to one side, her neck broken and her larynx collapsed, the old man's fingers with their frenzied power crushing the fragile cartilages and snapping the bones. And there was Old Jacob in the turbulent night with the rain pouring down on his head, the river loud, rushing, hurling itself against the old man, and Old Jacob fighting the swiftness, his angry face gaunt and lonely above the black water that pulled at him, his eyes fierce and hot.

You can't fight the swiftness of the river, Alex thought. It pulls at you and sucks you under with its contorted power. It eats away slowly, almost unseen, and then everything crumbles and dissolves into its swiftness. He saw Old Jacob fighting the river, never giving in, his arms beating wildly, groping, splashing, his hair plastered against his skull. He saw the terrible fury of his bony face.

The words that Moench had spoken to Alex kept coming back to him. He heard Moench's voice and he could still see the look in his eyes: "A man in destroying others, destroys himself."

Yes, Old Jacob must have known, must have been aware of the river bearing down on him in a terrible rush of water, and he allowed its cold rage to possess him.

~

*T*hose early months with Ellen arrested the wild fear that had gripped Alex. He succumbed completely to his new role as bridegroom. He began taking long brisk walks through the countryside, comparing the spring blossoms that hung heavy in the air with the perfume in Ellen's hair. Everything he saw and felt reminded him of Ellen. Deep in his mind, he continually saw the image of Liesa, who was so much like Ellen in every way. He was thrilled with every manifestation of spring. Underlying the happiness that seemed to overwhelm him was the sadness of what he considered his lost and lonely youth. He spent long hours convincing himself that he had found the one element capable of catalyzing him back into action in the laboratory. He was determined not to lose Ellen. This, he realized, was his last chance. Gradually, the images of Liesa and Ellen merged in his mind.

Underneath all this happiness, peering at him like some monstrous toad ready to pounce on him, was his old fear of the magic lamp.

He worked on the dialyzer with some of his former fierce intensity. After Hendricks became his assistant, he gradually became aware of a new corrosion overcoming him. Ellen's visits to the lab had been rare until his new assistant came. After his arrival, she began driving Alex to work. She'd come down for lunch and in the evening would pick him up again. At first, he had been pleased by this attention. More and more, he found himself detained by administrative details and Hendricks and Ellen would go off to lunch without him. It was odd with what frequency he was left behind at the lab, almost as if it had been planned. It seemed that Hendricks always managed to find some paper work or telephone calls for him to work on just at the moment Ellen arrived. At home, in the evening, Ellen could talk only of Hendricks; how beautifully he played the cello, how widely read he was, his knowledge of everything on the earth limitless.

All of Alex's old fears returned with renewed force. The old malignancy spread rapidly now. He began to examine the lamp in his study with greater intensity and frequency. It did not fragment and he felt moderately relieved.

He began to go to ignominious lengths to attract Ellen's attention. He wore a more youthful cut of clothes. Bright paisleys replaced his ancient ties. His visits to the barber became more frequent. He underwent elaborate hot mudpacks and special massages to strengthen his sagging facial muscles. He worked out in a "body shop" every other day. His falling hair bothered him and he combed it carefully to cover the bald areas. He applied Rogaine to his scalp religiously, after using a vibrator.

He took Ellen to expensive night clubs and tried to interest himself in the many superficialities that occupied her mind. He danced the latest dances with her and even lowered himself to attend rock concerts, which he detested passionately. Only individuals her own age were invited to their home.

He preferred to overlook the amused glances of his colleagues and frequently was heard to utter that hackneyed phrase: "You're only as old as you feel," while trying to ignore the osteoarthritic pains in his neck and back.

He was soon mouthing ideas on poetry, sculpture, and paintings, repeating witty and devastating criticisms of modern literature, bubbling over with false enthusiasm over the dissonant cacophony of serious modern music, and adapting mannerisms that were distinctly foreign to him. His friends snickered behind his back about his quick descent into senility, but partially forgave him because of his young wife and her influence on him. He spent less and less time at the lab, leaving his work on the dialyzer unfinished.

Ellen gradually looked at him with open contempt. This only made him try harder to excite her admiration. He was appalled at how quickly their relationship had deteriorated. When he began speaking about some matter concerning the creative arts, she would laugh at him derisively.

One day after one of his clumsy attempts at conversation, trying desperately to find some common ground with Ellen, she actually sneered at him.

"You'll never be another Jack Hendricks," she said laughing, "so why do you insist on making an old fool of yourself imitating him?"

Her lower lip curled in utter disdain.

Then it struck him for the first time in full force, this grotesque degeneration of his and the humiliating depths to which he had fallen. He wandered from the room dazed, unable to think, his world torn apart, uprooted, and totally disorganized.

With explosive force then, he was jarred back to the reality of his laboratory, his instruments, his animals, his work on the dialyzer. He had been an old man lost in a maze, accidentally stumbling into the correct passage that led the way out.

He moved a bed into the laboratory and worked feverishly to complete his data on the artificial kidney. He ignored Hendricks completely. He didn't see Ellen for weeks at a time. Perhaps this interlude of foolishness, he thought, was the exact stimulus he needed. He ate snacks, slept poorly an hour or two at a time, omitted shaving, and drove himself relentlessly within the bare, practical, functional sanctuary of the laboratory. And in his mind, partially suppressed by his renewed determination, was his old fear lurking behind every move he made. He worked in a mad frenzy to prevent its engulfing him.

Finally, his work was completed and he presented his paper at an international renal conference in New York. He exhibited the actual model of the portable dialyzer he had worked on for the last twenty years and discussed its unique ability to be used as an artificial kidney while the patient remained active. The enthusiasm with which it was received overwhelmed him and he could hardly contain his own joy.

If only Moench could have lived long enough to see this. If only Liesa could have been by his side. This is what I've worked for, he thought. All those years in the laboratory were not wasted. He saw the interested faces of the physicians in the huge hall, individuals from all over the world, listening to him speak, asking him complicated questions, consulting him on the various aspects of electrolyte therapy. They were the proof that his thirty-two years of hard work and sacrifice had paid off.

But something was missing. This great moment was not enough. There was no one to share his happiness. He felt an overpowering urge to talk to Ellen. He couldn't stay away from her any longer, even though they had drifted apart. She had remained at home in Connecticut with some vague malaise that had developed at the last moment.

He left the conference a day early and caught a train back to New Haven where he had left his car. He was somewhat startled to see that the rest of the world had not changed in any way, as he turned onto the ramp for Interstate 91 North. It took him about thirty minutes to reach his home. It was midnight and he thought of Ellen with her face clean against the pillow, asleep. He had forgotten about all her little nasty remarks that had made him feel so upset. He forgave her because of her youthful impetuosity. It takes a mature woman to understand an old man. It was his fault for marrying a mere child.

He saw a car parked up the street and on an impulse drove up to it to see the plate number. It was 488777. He felt a sudden tightening in his throat. He parked his car around the corner and walked slowly back to the house, his legs tired and dragging. It was completely dark. He tried the door and found it locked. He went around to the side of the house, walking on the soft wet grass. He stood in the darkness for a while outside the master bedroom windows on the first floor. Everything was quiet. He was about to leave when he heard the sounds, the voices, soft murmurs exploding in his ears. He walked carefully back to the front porch and waited in the shadows. It seemed a long time. Finally, he heard the door open and a dark figure came quickly down the steps.

He recognized that confident walk, almost a swagger, hands in his pockets, with the neck thrust forward slightly. He didn't have to see the face.

He stood in the darkness motionless, hearing the motor kick over and the car pulling away. He walked slowly up the front steps and opened the door quietly with the key. He stepped carefully to the bedroom door and gently opened it.

He heard Ellen turn over in bed and saw her raise herself on one elbow.

"I'm glad you decided to come back, Jack," she whispered hoarsely.

~

*H*e sat on his shivering horse and looked at the house, Old Jacob's House, what was left of it. He smelled the dankness of the rotting timbers. He could see no lights. He was rigid, hardly breathing. A deep cold filled his body. He could hear nothing but the pounding rain.

A cry ripped through the darkness, high, piercing, agonizing. He thought it would never end. He began to run, faster and faster. He heard the scream again, followed by a horrible sucking sound. He slipped on the grass and righted himself, arms swinging, his muscles aching with stiffness, his face hot with the cold rain beating against it. He wrenched open the massive oak door, the cry still ripping through the night. The door slammed shut behind him. He found himself in a well-lighted room. A slender dignified old man with a white beard stood tending a fire in the fireplace. He looked vaguely familiar. The old man turned around slowly and looked at Alex without saying a word. For a moment, Alex didn't know what to say.

"Who are you?" Alex finally blurted out. "You look familiar. Are you Old Jacob?"

"You come barging into my house demanding to know who I am," the old man said. "You are an impertinent rascal, sir. Leave this house immediately."

"Who are you?" Alex repeated, not moving a muscle.

"I am who I am," the old man answered, the fire poker still in his hand. "What are you doing here?"

"I received an emergency call about thirty minutes ago. I was told someone was dying. Now are you going to tell me who you are?"

"I am whoever you want me to be," the old man said. "And furthermore, you're too late."

Alex stood looking at the old man silently. He was confused.

"Are you my father?" Alex finally said.

"I could be your father if you want me to be."

"Is this some kind of riddle, some grand joke that you're playing on me?" Alex asked. "If it is, I certainly don't appreciate it. I could be home sleeping in my nice warm bed."

"We all could be in our beds or our graves if you hadn't come," the old man said.

"Are you here because of me?" Alex asked.

"Yes," the old man answered. "And you're here because of me."

"You are talking in riddles, old man," Alex said, impatient and angry. "Is this a dream, a nightmare?"

"It could be," the old man said, "if you want it to be."

Alex hesitated.

"Is my mother here?" he finally asked, not wanting to hear the answer.

"Yes."

"Where?"

"She's dead," the old man said.

"Did you kill her?" Alex asked.

"Yes," the old man said coldly. "She deserved to die. She was a whore."

Alex sat down and cried. If he had come sooner, he knew he could have saved her.

~

*T*he night Alex came back home early, he went into the study. Neither he nor Ellen spoke to each other.

He sat down and stared at the lamp on the table for an hour without shifting his gaze. It began to fragment finally, separating into many pieces, just as the lamp did in Austria. It took on an existence totally independent of time and place. He knew that he was entering an alien world again, where the real becomes unreal and the unreal becomes real. He was not afraid and felt rather indifferent about the whole matter. He heard voices again, drifting towards him from the wall, but they were uttering unintelligible sounds, a babble that he couldn't comprehend. He burst out laughing. He laughed harder and harder until he was breathless. He felt himself leave the room, propelled by some unearthly strange mechanism into outer space, millions of miles away, finally stopping near the Big Red Spot of Jupiter. He looked back at Earth and saw himself sitting in the chair, staring at the lamp. What a dreary, pitiful old man, dull, senseless, an individual obviously in the embrace of the devil. Why else would he stare at a lamp and watch it so carefully while the devil took it apart. The old man was obviously mesmerized. What a joy to be finally separated from him.

While he watched the old man in silent amusement, listening to nothing but the ghostly sound of the solar wind, he saw him go into a spasm and fall out of the chair. He jerked about wildly, all his muscles moving in rhythmic contractions, his extremities flailing about madly. He was frothing at the mouth with his teeth clenched tightly, snorting as he tried to breathe. His whole body was trembling, shivering, shaking. It seemed to Alex that the devil's seizure would never release the old man from its grip.

A priest in all his glorious vestments appeared and leaned over the old man. He held a gleaming gold cross aimed at the writhing figure on the floor. Alex heard the priest speaking, forceful, booming words, reverberating like thunder rolling across the universe:

"I adjure thee, O Serpent of Old, by the Judge of the living and dead; by the Creator of the World who hath power to cast into Hell, that thou depart forthwith from this house. He that commandeth thee, accursed demon, is He that commanded the winds, and the sea and the storm. He that commands thee, is He that ordered thee to be hurled down from the height of heaven into the lower parts of the earth. He that commands thee is He that bade thee depart from Him. Hearken then, Satan and fear. Get thee gone, vanquished and cowed, when thou art bidden in the name of our Lord Jesus Christ who will judge the living and the dead by fire. Amen."

As Alex heard the words in outer space, he started his journey back to earth. A quiet, peaceful serenity overtook him. As the priest uttered the final words of the exorcism, Alex opened his eyes.

It was hot and he couldn't move. A heavy weight seemed to be resting on his chest. He tried to raise himself to see his legs but couldn't and he lay there sweating and trembling in the darkness, afraid.

"Ellen," he called out.

All he could hear was the rain outside and he gradually became senseless to that. Everything was quiet. An unusual calm permeated the room. He could feel the sweat on his body like a million ants crawling, but he couldn't feel his arms and legs and the sweat didn't bother him there. The wind had died down and the night was like hot wool against his skin. The air was suffocating.

"Ellen," he yelled out again.

He turned his head but could see nothing. He thought he had become blind. He wanted to cry. He looked about rapidly, turning his head from side to side in a panic, but there was nothing but blackness.

"Ellen."

He bellowed this time, crying, his voice distorted by his trembling lips. He breathed very quickly. He felt the smooth boards of the floor as he moved his body. His mouth was dry and he kept licking his lips. He felt a sharp pain in his mouth where he had bitten his tongue.

He heard voices and footsteps on the stones of the path leading to the house. He lay in the darkness and listened.

It is Jacob, he thought, and someone is with him.

He heard the click of a flashlight and saw the beam outside the porch window. The boards of the floor creaked as a shrouded figure came in. He lay quietly and waited. The beam of the flashlight fell on his eyes and he blinked.

"Ellen," he said alarmed. "What are you doing out here on River Road? Where is Old Jacob?"

The flashlight clattered to the floor, the beam cutting across the room at a low angle. He saw Ellen looking at him, her face startled and her eyes glinting in the light.

"The River Road?" Ellen said, her voice harsh. "What are you talking about? Who is Jacob?"

He saw only the mouth move. The words seemed to come from everywhere. He tried to get up but he was too weak, his arms aching with the effort.

"Where's Hendricks?" he said.

Ellen picked up the flashlight and placed it on the table pointing away from them.

"Where's Hendricks?" he yelled, his voice tremulous and high.

Ellen turned away.

"Where's Hendricks, do you hear me, Ellen? Where is he? I demand to know. Something is terribly wrong. I can hardly move my arms and legs. Switch on the lights, for God's sake."

"The power's off," Ellen said, her voice flat. "The storm tore down the lines."

"Where's Hendricks? Where is he?"

"He's outside," Ellen said.

"Outside? Why is he outside?"

"We're leaving," Ellen said. "I've packed my bags. They're on the porch."

"You're lying, damn you," he screamed. "I'll never let you go."

Ellen moved closer.

"I just came in to tell you we're leaving tonight."

Now he remembered the telephone call, the voice hissing and telling him to hurry to the last house on River Road, Jacob's House.

"You're the one," he yelled. "You called me to come out here. You're the whore I killed in Austria."

He reached out and grabbed Ellen by the throat, dragging her screaming to the floor.

"Why didn't you die the first time I killed you and threw you into the river?" Alex screamed, snarling. "You're the whore."

He heard Ellen gasp as he pressed his thumbs hard against her larynx. He felt her arms flap about wildly. There was a loud snap and a horrible sucking sound. Her arms didn't beat so wildly as Ellen fell limp and heavy against him, hands clutching her throat.

The rain made a light tapping sound against the windows, while a tree somewhere, bending with the wind, scraped against the side of the house.

He kept his eyes closed and lay there shaking, the sweat heavy on his body. After a while, he was surprised to feel the smoothness of the leather couch beneath him. He thought he had been on the floor. He slid his fingers along its coolness, its slickness. He turned his head and smelled the leather and he wasn't afraid anymore. He thought of the familiar cabinets of his study, the shelves of books, the old roll-top desk. He felt his body loosen in his wet clothes. He was in his own home in the city, not in his country cabin. The River Road was miles away, a horrible part of his nightmare. He ached all over dully and a sharp pain shot in his mouth up to his right ear. He tasted blood in his mouth and he felt like vomiting, but he just lay there on the couch quietly.

He heard the rain beating against the windows and the tree scraping against the house and he was afraid again. He saw the lamp on the table. It was fragmented, the individual pieces suspended in midair. He knew it would never be normal again.

He saw Old Jacob now, the contorted face above the black twisted water, the gaunt fury and the loneliness, the thick furrowed leather of the skin, the fierce eyes sunk deep into the bones of the skull, unblinking, blazing, masklike, the arms beating, hands clawing, fighting the swiftness of the river, his body twisting and writhing, and then being carried high upon the water that drew upon itself, lifted into the violent blackness of the sky in a terrible wave that shuddered and hung in the air for one prolonged moment, as if suspended by some invisible wires that suddenly snapped, the water then lipping over white and dropping heavily, crushing Jacob's torn body against the trunk of a tree, spreading out smooth, almost motionless, and then rushing on with a horrible sucking sound, like a long drawn-out human gasp, the final desolate wrenching cry from the swelling throat lost in the haunting wind and the furious confusion of trembling leaves.

"Father," Alex whispered hoarsely. "It's Alex, your son. I've come home and I forgive you."

He opened his eyes and the room spun dizzily. He turned quickly and saw the flashlight on the table. Then the door was flung open and he saw Hendricks standing in front of him with horror in his eyes.

He looked down quickly and saw Ellen sprawled on the floor, her head turned back at a weird angle.

Lessons To Be Learned

Dr. Alex Honicutt and I discussed the tragic story of his life two weeks before he died at a hospital for the criminally insane, where he had been incarcerated for the previous five years. Authorities stated he had fallen on the stairs and sustained a fracture of his cervical spine with transection of his spinal cord. I assumed he had been killed by one of the other violent inmates at the institution.

My friendship with Dr. Honicutt dated back to our college days even though we had never been close. He was a loner and preferred a relative isolation. This is not an unusual premorbid personality in individuals who develop schizophrenia. Dr. Honicutt, despite his brilliance, had no faith in psychiatry and never sought help of any kind. This attitude is not uncommon among physicians. One of the reasons behind this attitude, of course, is that all antipsychotic medications can cause serious side effects. Dr. Honicutt had a mission in life which he carried out successfully. He may not have been able to do so under the influence of the various drugs used in this condition.

Because he was in research, he posed no danger to patients. However, there are physicians suffering from schizophrenia who are actively taking care of patients in private practice. Obviously, they are in a position to do great harm. Recently, a surgeon made the headlines in another state. While doing a simple prostatectomy, he went on to excise the bladder and disembowel the patient before he could be stopped. The patient died. After only a brief period of psychiatric treatment, this surgeon was allowed to return to the private practice of surgery, supposedly under supervision. His license to practice was never taken away.

Schizophrenia is a grave disorder of the mind and personality that seriously impairs an individual's ability to comprehend reality. It is such a terrible commotion of thought processes, such a wild tumult of moods and aberrations that it becomes almost incomprehensible to a normal person.

The most common diagnostic features of this condition are auditory and visual hallucinations, which are false sensory perceptions, and delusions, which are beliefs that have no basis in reality.

The onset can be so insidious that it goes unnoticed, or so explosive that it immediately becomes a media event. Usually the more abrupt the onset, the quicker the return to the premorbid state, or nearly so, frequently without any residual changes in the afflicted individual.

There are no pathological changes in the brain associated with schizophrenia and most schizophrenics have no recognizable premorbid personalities, even though some are relatively isolated loners as I've already mentioned. These patients may appear entirely normal in between attacks or progress to a state that demands immediate intervention.

The auditory hallucinations most commonly take the form of hearing one's thoughts or hearing remarks of one or two voices commenting on the individual himself or his activities.

The most common delusion is that of a super-powerful force that has taken complete control of the patient through radio waves compelling him to react in abnormal ways.

The schizophrenic may appear remote, indifferent, and cold. His emotional reactions can be punctuated by sudden bursts of incongruent laughter entirely unrelated to the thoughts he is expressing. At the same time he may exhibit athetoid motions (sinuous, writhing motions) or appear stuporous and catatonic. Chronic amphetamine intoxication can simulate the signs and symptoms of schizophrenia with marked restlessness, fits of anger, and extreme anxiety, associated with a rambling, disjointed speech. Some epileptics may exhibit a state resembling schizophrenia with associated paranoia, auditory hallucinations and delusions. Chronically inebriated individuals suddenly withdrawing from alcohol can display similar aberrant thought processes associated with hallucinations, delusions, and even hypoglycemia.

Antipsychotic drugs can be categorized by their ability to block dopamine receptors, dopamine being a compound found in cerebral tissue. The stronger drugs also have serious side effects such as motor restlessness (akathesia), dystonia (disorganized muscle motion) and parkinsonian symptoms. These drugs may also precipitate neuroleptic malignant syndrome (NMS) characterized by a deterioration of consciousness, hyperthermia, and muscle rigidity with a death rate as high as 30%. Another disturbing side effect of some of these drugs is tardive dyskinesia presenting as involuntary movements of the tongue, lips, face, and mouth.

One of the newer drugs is Clozaril, which not only blocks dopamine receptors, but also serotonin receptors. It too, may cause serious side effects and may not be effective in every patient.

Schizophrenia is, therefore, a disorder of the mind which exhibits a wild, incomprehensible mixture of the bizarre, the grotesque, the incongruent, intermixed with periods of complete lucidity.

Alex Honicutt was aware of his ultimate intellectual deterioration. Because he visualized himself as a man with a mission and was aware of the consequences of drug therapy, he opted to go it alone, fearing that the treatment, in his case, could be worse than the brain disorder he suffered, preventing him completely from continuing his work on the portable dialyzer. After all, in between his infrequent attacks, he regained his premorbid state and was able to return to his laboratory and the only work that mattered to him.

Eventually, however, the final explosive episode forced his incarceration and subsequently his death, which I suspected, as I mentioned before, was probably at the hands of another inmate.

Is a patient capable of recognizing schizoid tendencies in a physician?

Probably not. Of course, if the doctor's actions, personality, and mood are bizarre enough, these changes could be recognized by anybody. But the schizophrenic individual is by no means stupid. He is usually aware that he perceives reality in a much different way than the ordinary person. He also knows that other people are not receiving the same messages that seem to be entering his brain electronically.

He is fully capable of suppressing any abnormalities, while presenting himself as a perfectly healthy, lucid individual.

He can even fool a psychiatrist.